THE DIABETIC COOKBOOK FOR NEWLY DIAGNOSED

A Beginner's Guide To 2000 Delicious Days Of Super Easy And Healthy Diabetics Diet Recipes With Complete Food List And Meal Planner For Type 1 & 2 Diabetes

Nathan Wendy

Table of Contents

CHAPTER ONE 5
Understanding Diabetes and Nutrition 5
What is Diabetes and How Does It Affect Diet? 5
The Role of Carbohydrates, Proteins, and Fats in Blood Sugar Control 7
Reading Food Labels and Understanding Nutritional Information 8

CHAPTER TWO 10
Essential Tools and Ingredients for Diabetic Cooking 10
Stocking Your Pantry with Diabetic-Friendly Staples 10
Must-Have Kitchen Equipment for Easy Diabetic Cooking 12
Understanding Sweeteners and Substitutes 13

CHAPTER THREE 16
Breakfasts to Start Your Day Right 16
Quick and Nutritious Breakfast Options for Busy Mornings 16
High-Fiber Breakfasts to Keep You Full and Energized 17
Diabetic-Friendly Smoothie and Oatmeal Recipes 19

CHAPTER FOUR 21
Healthy and Flavorful Lunches 21
Simple Salad and Sandwich Ideas for Diabetic Lunches 21

Protein-Packed Lunches to Satisfy Hunger and Stabilize Blood Sugar 22

CHAPTER FIVE 25

Wholesome Dinners for Every Palate 25

Easy One-Pan Dinners for Minimal Cleanup 25

Comforting Slow Cooker and Instant Pot Recipes 28

CHAPTER SIX 30

Smart Snacks for Between Meals 30

Nutrient-Dense Snack Ideas to Keep Blood Sugar Stable 30

Homemade Snacks That Are Low in Added Sugar and High in Flavor 31

Portable Snacks for On-the-Go Convenience 33

CHAPTER SEVEN 35

Delectable Desserts Without the Guilt 35

Lower-Sugar Dessert Recipes for Sweet Cravings 35

CHAPTER EIGHT 39

Flavorful Side Dishes to Accompany Any Meal 39

Simple Vegetable Side Dishes Packed with Nutrients 39

Whole Grain and Legume-Based Side Dishes for Sustained Energy 40

Creative Ways to Add Flavor to Your Side Dish Repertoire 41

CHAPTER NINE 44

Entertaining and Special Occasion Menus 44

Hosting a Diabetic-Friendly Dinner Party or Gathering 44

Special Occasion Menus That Wow Without Compromising Health 47

CHAPTER TEN 87

Meal Planning and Prepping for Success 87

Strategies for Efficient Meal Planning and Grocery Shopping . 87

Batch Cooking and Freezing Meals for Convenience 88

Tips for Maintaining a Balanced Diet and Managing Portions . 90

CHAPTER 11 104

DIET FOR DIABETES 104

CHAPTER 12 149

31 DAYS MEAL PLAN 149

THE END 159

COPYRIGHT © 2023

All rights reserved. No part of this publication may be reproduced, distributed, or transmitted in any form or by any means, including photocopying, recording, or other electronic or mechanical methods, without the prior written permission of the publisher, except in the case of brief quotations embodied in critical reviews and certain other noncommercial uses permitted by copyright law.

CHAPTER ONE

Understanding Diabetes and Nutrition

What is Diabetes and How Does It Affect Diet?

Diabetes is a chronic condition characterized by high levels of glucose (sugar) in the blood. It occurs when the body either doesn't produce enough insulin or can't effectively use the insulin it produces. Insulin is a hormone produced by the pancreas that helps regulate blood sugar levels and allows glucose to enter cells, where it can be used for energy.

There are two main types of diabetes: type 1 and type 2. Type 1 diabetes typically develops during childhood or adolescence and is an autoimmune condition where the body's immune system mistakenly attacks and destroys the insulin-producing cells in the pancreas. As a result, people with type 1 diabetes require insulin injections to survive.

Type 2 diabetes, on the other hand, is more common and often develops in adulthood, although it is increasingly being diagnosed in children and adolescents due to rising obesity rates. In type 2 diabetes, the body becomes resistant to the effects of insulin or doesn't produce enough insulin to maintain normal blood sugar levels.

Regardless of the type, managing diabetes involves making healthy lifestyle choices, including following a balanced diet. Diet plays a crucial role in diabetes management because the foods we eat directly impact blood sugar levels. By understanding how different nutrients affect blood sugar and making informed food choices, individuals with diabetes can better control their condition and reduce the risk of complications.

For people with diabetes, it's important to focus on eating a variety of nutrient-rich foods in appropriate portions to help regulate blood sugar levels, maintain a healthy weight, and prevent other health problems associated with diabetes, such as heart disease and nerve damage.

The Role of Carbohydrates, Proteins, and Fats in Blood Sugar Control

Carbohydrates, proteins, and fats are the three macronutrients that make up the bulk of our diet and have distinct roles in blood sugar control.

Carbohydrates: Carbohydrates are the body's primary source of energy, and they have the greatest impact on blood sugar levels. When carbohydrates are digested, they are broken down into glucose, which enters the bloodstream and raises blood sugar levels. Therefore, people with diabetes need to be mindful of their carbohydrate intake and choose carbohydrates that have a minimal impact on blood sugar, such as whole grains, fruits, vegetables, and legumes. They should also pay attention to portion sizes and spacing out carbohydrate-containing foods throughout the day to prevent spikes in blood sugar.

Proteins: Proteins are essential for building and repairing tissues in the body, including muscles, organs, and skin. Unlike carbohydrates, proteins have a minimal effect on blood sugar levels when consumed in moderate amounts. However, large amounts of protein can still stimulate insulin secretion and affect blood sugar, so it's important to include protein-rich foods in moderation as part of a balanced diet. Good sources of protein for people with diabetes include lean meats, poultry, fish, eggs, tofu, nuts, and seeds.

Fats: Fats are another important source of energy and play a role in nutrient absorption, hormone production, and cell function. While fats do not directly affect blood sugar levels, they can influence insulin sensitivity and overall health. Saturated and trans fats, found in foods such as red meat, butter, and fried foods, can increase the risk of heart disease and should be limited in the diet. On the other hand, unsaturated fats, found in foods such as olive oil, avocado, and nuts, can have beneficial effects on heart health when consumed in moderation.

Reading Food Labels and Understanding Nutritional Information

Reading food labels and understanding nutritional information is essential for making informed choices about the foods we eat, especially for people with diabetes who need to monitor their carbohydrate intake and manage blood sugar levels.

Ingredients List: The ingredients list on a food label provides valuable information about the contents of a product. Ingredients are listed in descending order by weight, so the first ingredient listed is present in the highest amount. People with diabetes should look for products with whole, minimally processed ingredients and avoid foods with added sugars, refined grains, and unhealthy fats.

Nutrition Facts Panel: The nutrition facts panel on a food label provides detailed information about the nutrient content of a product, including serving size, calories, macronutrients (carbohydrates, proteins, and fats), vitamins, minerals, and other important nutrients. When reading the nutrition facts panel, it's important to pay attention to serving sizes and the total amount of carbohydrates, especially sugars and fiber, as well as other nutrients that may affect blood sugar levels, such as sodium.

Carbohydrate Counting: Carbohydrate counting is a method used by people with diabetes to track their carbohydrate intake and manage blood sugar levels. It involves estimating the amount of carbohydrates in foods based on their portion size and carbohydrate content, as indicated on food labels. By keeping track of their carbohydrate intake and adjusting their insulin doses or mealtime medications accordingly, people with diabetes can better control their blood sugar levels and optimize their overall health.

In conclusion, understanding diabetes and nutrition is essential for effectively managing the condition and preventing complications. By following a balanced diet that focuses on nutrient-rich foods, monitoring carbohydrate intake, and making informed choices based on food labels and nutritional information, people with diabetes can improve their blood sugar control, reduce the risk of complications, and lead healthier lives.

CHAPTER TWO

Essential Tools and Ingredients for Diabetic Cooking

Stocking Your Pantry with Diabetic-Friendly Staples

Maintaining a well-stocked pantry with diabetic-friendly staples is key to making healthy and delicious meals at home. Here are some essential ingredients to consider:

Whole Grains: Whole grains are rich in fiber and complex carbohydrates, which help regulate blood sugar levels and promote overall health. Stock up on options like brown rice, quinoa, oats, barley, and whole wheat pasta to incorporate into your meals.

Legumes: Beans, lentils, and chickpeas are excellent sources of protein, fiber, and essential nutrients. They have a low glycemic index, meaning they cause a gradual rise in blood sugar levels, making them ideal for people with diabetes. Canned or dried varieties are convenient options to keep in your pantry for quick and nutritious meals.

Healthy Fats: Opt for heart-healthy fats such as olive oil, avocado oil, nuts, seeds, and nut butters. These fats provide essential nutrients and can help improve insulin sensitivity and reduce the risk of heart disease.

Non-Starchy Vegetables: Fill your pantry with a variety of non-starchy vegetables like spinach, kale, broccoli, bell peppers, cauliflower, and tomatoes. These vegetables are low in carbohydrates and calories but high in fiber, vitamins, and minerals, making them perfect for managing blood sugar levels and promoting satiety.

Canned Tomatoes and Tomato Products: Canned tomatoes, tomato paste, and tomato sauce are versatile ingredients that add flavor and depth to dishes without the need for added sugars. Look for options without added salt or sugar for a healthier choice.

Herbs and Spices: Herbs and spices are essential for adding flavor to meals without extra calories, sodium, or sugar. Keep a variety of options on hand, such as garlic, ginger, basil, oregano, cinnamon, and turmeric, to enhance the taste of your dishes.

Low-Sodium Broth or Stock: Stocking your pantry with low-sodium broth or stock is a convenient way to add flavor to soups, stews, and sauces without excess salt. Look for options made from vegetables, chicken, or beef and check the label for added sugars and artificial ingredients.

Must-Have Kitchen Equipment for Easy Diabetic Cooking

Having the right kitchen equipment can make diabetic cooking more efficient and enjoyable. Here are some essential tools to consider:

Quality Chef's Knife: A sharp chef's knife is essential for chopping, dicing, and slicing ingredients with precision. Invest in a high-quality knife that feels comfortable in your hand and maintains its sharpness over time.

Cutting Board: Choose a durable cutting board made from wood, plastic, or bamboo that provides a stable surface for prepping ingredients. Consider having multiple cutting boards to prevent cross-contamination between raw meats, vegetables, and other foods.

Non-Stick Cookware: Non-stick pots and pans are ideal for cooking with minimal oil or fat, reducing the need for added calories and unhealthy fats. Look for pots and pans with a durable non-stick coating that can withstand high temperatures and regular use.

Measuring Cups and Spoons: Accurately measuring ingredients is crucial for achieving consistent results in diabetic cooking. Invest in a set of measuring cups and spoons for dry and liquid ingredients to ensure portion control and balanced meals.

Food Scale: A digital food scale is a valuable tool for portion control and accurate measuring, especially when it comes to carbohydrate counting and managing blood sugar levels. Use the food scale to weigh ingredients like grains, meats, and produce for precise cooking and meal planning.

Slow Cooker or Instant Pot: Slow cookers and Instant Pots are versatile appliances that make meal preparation a breeze. They allow you to cook a variety of dishes, from soups and stews to whole grains and lean proteins, with minimal hands-on time. These appliances are particularly useful for busy individuals who want to enjoy healthy, home-cooked meals without spending hours in the kitchen.

Understanding Sweeteners and Substitutes

Choosing the right sweeteners and substitutes is important for managing blood sugar levels and reducing the intake of added sugars in the diet. Here are some options to consider:

Natural Sweeteners: Natural sweeteners like stevia, monk fruit extract, and erythritol are low-calorie alternatives to sugar that do not raise blood sugar levels. These sweeteners can be used in moderation to add sweetness to beverages, baked goods, and other recipes without affecting blood sugar control.

Artificial Sweeteners: Artificial sweeteners like aspartame, sucralose, and saccharin are calorie-free sugar substitutes that provide sweetness without affecting blood sugar levels. While they are safe for most people with diabetes, some individuals may experience gastrointestinal discomfort or other side effects, so it's important to use them in moderation and monitor how your body responds.

Sugar Alcohols: Sugar alcohols like xylitol, sorbitol, and mannitol are carbohydrates that provide sweetness without causing a rapid increase in blood sugar levels. However, they can have a laxative effect and may cause digestive issues in some people, especially when consumed in large amounts.

Fruit Purees: Fruit purees made from mashed bananas, applesauce, or dates can be used as natural sweeteners in recipes like baked goods, sauces, and dressings. They add sweetness, moisture, and flavor without the need for added sugars or artificial sweeteners.

Portion Control: Regardless of the type of sweetener used, it's important to practice portion control and moderation to prevent spikes in blood sugar levels. Even low-calorie or sugar-free sweeteners can contribute to excess calorie intake if consumed in large amounts.

In summary, stocking your pantry with diabetic-friendly staples, investing in essential kitchen equipment, and understanding sweeteners and substitutes are key components of successful diabetic cooking. By incorporating nutritious ingredients, using the right tools, and making smart choices about sweeteners, individuals with diabetes can enjoy delicious meals that support their health and well-being.

CHAPTER THREE

Breakfasts to Start Your Day Right

Quick and Nutritious Breakfast Options for Busy Mornings

Breakfast is often hailed as the most important meal of the day, but busy mornings can make it challenging to prepare a nutritious meal. Here are some quick and convenient breakfast options to fuel your day:

Greek Yogurt Parfait: Layer Greek yogurt with fresh or frozen berries, nuts, and a drizzle of honey or maple syrup for a protein-rich and satisfying breakfast. Greek yogurt is high in protein and probiotics, which promote gut health and keep you feeling full until your next meal.

Whole Grain Toast with Nut Butter: Spread whole grain toast with almond butter, peanut butter, or sunflower seed butter for a simple and filling breakfast. Top with sliced bananas, strawberries, or chia seeds for added flavor and nutrition. Whole grain bread provides fiber and complex carbohydrates, while nut butter adds healthy fats and protein.

Overnight Oats: Prepare overnight oats by combining rolled oats with milk or yogurt, chia seeds, and your choice of sweeteners and flavorings in a jar or container. Let the mixture sit in the refrigerator overnight, and enjoy it cold or warmed up in the morning. Overnight oats are customizable and can be topped with fruits, nuts, seeds, or spices for added texture and flavor.

Egg Muffins: Whip up a batch of egg muffins ahead of time and store them in the refrigerator or freezer for a quick and portable breakfast option. Simply beat eggs with your favorite vegetables, cheese, and seasonings, pour the mixture into muffin tins, and bake until set. Egg muffins are high in protein and can be customized to suit your taste preferences.

High-Fiber Breakfasts to Keep You Full and Energized

Fiber is an essential nutrient that promotes digestive health, regulates blood sugar levels, and keeps you feeling full and satisfied. Incorporating high-fiber foods into your breakfast can help you stay energized throughout the morning. Here are some ideas:

Whole Grain Cereal with Fruit: Choose a high-fiber cereal made from whole grains and top it with fresh or dried fruit, nuts, and seeds for added fiber and nutrients. Look for cereals with at least 3 grams of fiber per serving and minimal added sugars. Serve with milk or yogurt for extra protein and calcium.

Chia Seed Pudding: Mix chia seeds with milk or a dairy-free alternative, such as almond milk or coconut milk, and let the mixture sit in the refrigerator until thickened. Stir in sweeteners and flavorings like vanilla extract, cinnamon, or cocoa powder, and top with berries, sliced fruit, or nuts. Chia seeds are packed with fiber, omega-3 fatty acids, and antioxidants, making them an excellent choice for a high-fiber breakfast.

Vegetable Omelette: Load up your omelette with fiber-rich vegetables like spinach, bell peppers, onions, tomatoes, and mushrooms for a nutritious and filling breakfast. Add a sprinkle of cheese or a dollop of avocado for extra flavor and satiety. Eggs are a good source of protein and essential nutrients, while vegetables provide fiber, vitamins, and minerals.

Whole Grain Pancakes or Waffles: Swap traditional pancakes or waffles for whole grain versions made with whole wheat flour, oat flour, or buckwheat flour. Serve with fresh fruit, Greek yogurt, or nut butter for added fiber and protein. Whole grain pancakes and waffles are hearty and satisfying, perfect for a leisurely weekend breakfast or meal prep for busy weekdays.

Diabetic-Friendly Smoothie and Oatmeal Recipes

Smoothies and oatmeal are popular breakfast options that can be easily customized to meet the dietary needs of people with diabetes. Here are some diabetic-friendly recipes to try:

Berry Blast Smoothie: Blend together frozen mixed berries, spinach, Greek yogurt, almond milk, and a splash of lemon juice for a refreshing and nutrient-rich smoothie. Berries are low in carbohydrates and high in fiber and antioxidants, making them an excellent choice for people with diabetes. Add a scoop of protein powder or a tablespoon of chia seeds for extra protein and fiber.

Cinnamon Apple Oatmeal: Cook rolled oats with unsweetened applesauce, cinnamon, and a pinch of salt until creamy and tender. Top with chopped apples, walnuts, and a drizzle of honey or maple syrup for sweetness. Cinnamon helps regulate blood sugar levels and adds warm, comforting flavor to the oatmeal.

This hearty and satisfying breakfast will keep you full and energized until lunchtime.

Green Smoothie Bowl: Blend together spinach, kale, banana, avocado, almond milk, and a scoop of protein powder until smooth and creamy. Pour the smoothie into a bowl and top with sliced kiwi, strawberries, granola, and a sprinkle of hemp seeds or flaxseeds. Green smoothie bowls are packed with vitamins, minerals, and fiber, making them an excellent choice for a nutritious and diabetic-friendly breakfast.

Pumpkin Spice Overnight Oats: Mix rolled oats with canned pumpkin puree, pumpkin pie spice, vanilla extract, and a sweetener of your choice, such as stevia or erythritol. Stir in almond milk or coconut milk until well combined, and let the mixture sit in the refrigerator overnight. In the morning, top the oats with chopped pecans, a dollop of Greek yogurt, and a drizzle of maple syrup for a festive and satisfying breakfast.

In conclusion, starting your day with a nutritious breakfast is essential for maintaining energy levels, managing blood sugar levels, and supporting overall health. Whether you prefer quick and convenient options for busy mornings, high-fiber choices to keep you full and satisfied, or diabetic-friendly smoothies and oatmeal recipes, there are plenty of delicious and satisfying breakfast options to choose from. Experiment with different ingredients and flavors to find what works best for you and enjoy a healthy start to your day.

CHAPTER FOUR

Healthy and Flavorful Lunches

Simple Salad and Sandwich Ideas for Diabetic Lunches

Salads and sandwiches are versatile lunch options that can be customized to suit your taste preferences and dietary needs. Here are some simple and nutritious ideas for diabetic-friendly lunches:

Grilled Chicken Caesar Salad: Toss grilled chicken breast slices with romaine lettuce, cherry tomatoes, cucumber slices, and a sprinkle of grated Parmesan cheese. Drizzle with a light Caesar dressing made with Greek yogurt, lemon juice, garlic, and Dijon mustard for a healthier twist on the classic salad.

Turkey and Avocado Wrap: Spread a whole grain tortilla with mashed avocado and top with sliced turkey breast, spinach leaves, shredded carrots, and bell pepper strips. Roll up the wrap tightly and slice it into pinwheels for a portable and satisfying lunch option. Turkey is a lean source of protein, while avocado adds healthy fats and fiber.

Mediterranean Veggie Sandwich: Layer whole grain bread with hummus, roasted red pepper strips, sliced cucumber, red onion, and Kalamata olives for a Mediterranean-inspired sandwich. Add a handful of baby spinach or arugula for extra greens and flavor. This sandwich is packed with fiber, vitamins, and minerals, making it a nutritious and satisfying meal.

Tuna Salad Lettuce Wraps: Mix canned tuna with Greek yogurt, diced celery, red onion, and a squeeze of lemon juice for a lighter version of classic tuna salad. Spoon the tuna salad into lettuce leaves and top with sliced avocado, cherry tomatoes, and sprouts for added crunch and freshness. Lettuce wraps are low in carbohydrates and calories, making them a great option for people with diabetes.

Protein-Packed Lunches to Satisfy Hunger and Stabilize Blood Sugar

Incorporating protein-rich foods into your lunch can help keep you feeling full and satisfied while stabilizing blood sugar levels. Here are some protein-packed lunch ideas to try:

Quinoa and Black Bean Salad: Combine cooked quinoa with black beans, diced bell peppers, corn kernels, cherry tomatoes, and chopped cilantro. Toss with a simple dressing made with lime juice, olive oil, cumin, and chili powder for a flavorful and filling salad. Quinoa and black beans are both excellent sources of plant-based protein and fiber.

Salmon and Vegetable Stir-Fry: Stir-fry salmon fillets with a variety of colorful vegetables like broccoli, bell peppers, snap peas, and carrots in a ginger-garlic sauce. Serve the stir-fry over cooked brown rice or cauliflower rice for a nutritious and satisfying meal. Salmon is rich in omega-3 fatty acids, which have been shown to reduce inflammation and improve insulin sensitivity.

Greek Yogurt Chicken Salad: Mix shredded cooked chicken breast with Greek yogurt, diced apples, grapes, celery, and walnuts for a creamy and protein-packed chicken salad. Season with a pinch of curry powder, salt, and pepper for added flavor. Serve the chicken salad over mixed greens or whole grain crackers for a balanced and satisfying lunch.

Egg and Vegetable Frittata: Whip up a vegetable frittata using eggs, egg whites, and a variety of chopped vegetables such as spinach, bell peppers, onions, and mushrooms. Bake the frittata in a skillet until set and golden brown, then slice it into wedges for an easy and portable lunch option. Eggs are a complete source of protein and contain essential nutrients like vitamin D and B vitamins.

Creative Lunchbox Ideas for Work or School

Packing a nutritious and delicious lunchbox is a great way to ensure you have a healthy meal on hand when you're on the go. Here are some creative lunchbox ideas to inspire you:

Bento Box with Hummus and Veggie Dippers: Fill a bento box with individual compartments with hummus, baby carrots, cucumber slices, cherry tomatoes, snap peas, and whole grain crackers for dipping. Include a small container of mixed nuts or trail mix for a crunchy and satisfying snack.

Mason Jar Salad: Layer a mason jar with salad ingredients like mixed greens, cherry tomatoes, shredded carrots, cucumber slices, and grilled chicken breast. Pack the dressing separately in a small container and toss everything together just before eating for a fresh and convenient salad on the go.

DIY Taco Salad Kit: Pack a divided container with lettuce leaves, seasoned ground turkey or tofu, black beans, diced avocado, salsa, shredded cheese, and tortilla strips. Assemble the taco salad by filling the lettuce leaves with the toppings and drizzling with lime juice for a portable and flavorful meal.

Sushi Roll Wraps: Roll up sushi ingredients like cooked brown rice, sliced cucumber, avocado, and cooked shrimp or tofu in nori sheets for a fun and nutritious lunch option. Serve with soy sauce, wasabi, and pickled ginger for dipping and extra flavor.

In summary, creating healthy and flavorful lunches doesn't have to be complicated. By incorporating nutrient-rich ingredients like lean proteins, whole grains, vegetables, and healthy fats into your meals, you can enjoy delicious and satisfying lunches that support your overall health and well-being. Experiment with different recipes and ingredients to keep your lunches exciting and enjoyable, whether you're eating at home, at work, or on the go.

CHAPTER FIVE

Wholesome Dinners for Every Palate

Easy One-Pan Dinners for Minimal Cleanup

One-pan dinners are perfect for busy weeknights when you want a delicious meal without the hassle of multiple pots and pans to clean up. Here are some easy and flavorful one-pan dinner ideas:

Sheet Pan Chicken and Vegetables: Arrange chicken breasts or thighs on a sheet pan with a variety of colorful vegetables like bell peppers, onions, zucchini, and cherry tomatoes. Drizzle with olive oil and season with your favorite herbs and spices, then roast in the oven until the chicken is cooked through and the vegetables are tender. Serve with cooked quinoa, brown rice, or whole grain pasta for a complete meal.

One-Pot Pasta Primavera: Cook whole wheat pasta in a large pot of boiling water until al dente, then add fresh or frozen vegetables like broccoli, peas, spinach, and cherry tomatoes to the pot during the last few minutes of cooking. Drain the pasta and vegetables, then toss with olive oil, garlic, lemon zest, and grated Parmesan cheese for a light and flavorful dinner that's ready in minutes.

Skillet Shrimp Stir-Fry: Sauté shrimp, bell peppers, snap peas, carrots, and broccoli in a large skillet with garlic, ginger, and soy sauce for a quick and healthy stir-fry. Serve over cooked brown rice or cauliflower rice for a low-carb option. Garnish with chopped green onions and sesame seeds for extra flavor and texture.

Quinoa Stuffed Bell Peppers: Cut the tops off bell peppers and remove the seeds and membranes. Fill the peppers with cooked quinoa mixed with black beans, corn, diced tomatoes, onions, and spices like cumin and chili powder. Bake in the oven until the peppers are tender and the filling is heated through. Top with shredded cheese and fresh cilantro before serving.

Flavorful Vegetarian and Plant-Based Dinner Options

Vegetarian and plant-based dinners are not only nutritious but also delicious and satisfying. Here are some flavorful options to try:

Vegetable Curry with Coconut Milk: Sauté onions, garlic, ginger, and curry paste in a large pot until fragrant, then add diced vegetables like potatoes, carrots, cauliflower, and bell peppers. Pour in coconut milk and vegetable broth, then simmer until the vegetables are tender and the flavors have melded together. Serve the curry over cooked brown rice or quinoa for a filling and comforting meal.

Chickpea and Spinach Masala: Simmer canned chickpeas in a spiced tomato sauce with onions, garlic, ginger, and garam masala until thick and flavorful. Stir in fresh spinach until wilted, then finish with a squeeze of lemon juice and a dollop of Greek yogurt for creaminess. Serve with naan bread or whole wheat pita for dipping.

Mushroom and Lentil Shepherd's Pie: Sauté onions, garlic, mushrooms, carrots, and celery in a skillet until softened, then add cooked lentils, tomato paste, Worcestershire sauce, and vegetable broth. Simmer until thickened, then transfer the mixture to a baking dish and top with mashed sweet potatoes or cauliflower. Bake in the oven until golden and bubbling. This hearty and comforting dish is perfect for a cozy night in.

Roasted Vegetable and Chickpea Buddha Bowl: Roast a variety of vegetables like sweet potatoes, Brussels sprouts, cauliflower, and red onions on a sheet pan until caramelized and tender. Toss cooked chickpeas with olive oil and spices like cumin and paprika, then roast until crispy. Serve the roasted vegetables and chickpeas over cooked quinoa or brown rice with a drizzle of tahini sauce and a sprinkle of fresh herbs for a nourishing and satisfying meal.

Comforting Slow Cooker and Instant Pot Recipes

Slow cooker and Instant Pot recipes are lifesavers for busy days when you want a hot and comforting meal with minimal effort. Here are some comforting options to try:

Slow Cooker Chili: Brown ground turkey or beef with onions, garlic, and spices like chili powder, cumin, and paprika in a skillet, then transfer to a slow cooker. Add canned tomatoes, tomato sauce, kidney beans, black beans, and diced bell peppers, then cook on low for 6-8 hours or high for 3-4 hours. Serve the chili topped with shredded cheese, Greek yogurt, and sliced green onions for a hearty and satisfying dinner.

Instant Pot Lentil Soup: Sauté onions, carrots, celery, and garlic in the Instant Pot until softened, then add dried lentils, canned diced tomatoes, vegetable broth, and spices like thyme and bay leaves. Cook on high pressure for 15 minutes, then release the pressure naturally. Stir in fresh spinach and lemon juice before serving. This comforting and nutritious soup is perfect for a chilly evening.

Slow Cooker Chicken and Vegetable Stew: Place chicken thighs or breasts in a slow cooker with chopped vegetables like potatoes, carrots, celery, and onions. Add chicken broth, garlic, thyme, and rosemary, then cook on low for 6-8 hours or high for 3-4 hours until the chicken is tender and the vegetables are cooked through. Serve the stew with crusty whole grain bread for dipping.

Instant Pot Butternut Squash Risotto: Sauté diced butternut squash, onions, and garlic in the Instant Pot until softened, then add Arborio rice and white wine and cook until the wine is absorbed. Stir in vegetable broth, thyme, and Parmesan cheese, then cook on high pressure for 6 minutes. Release the pressure naturally, then stir in baby spinach until wilted. This creamy and comforting risotto is perfect for a cozy night in.

In summary, wholesome dinners can be delicious, satisfying, and easy to prepare, whether you're cooking for yourself, your family, or guests. By incorporating a variety of nutritious ingredients like lean proteins, whole grains, vegetables, and plant-based foods into your meals, you can create flavorful dishes that appeal to every palate and support your health and well-being. Experiment with different recipes, flavors, and cooking techniques to keep your dinners exciting and enjoyable, and don't forget to savor each bite.

CHAPTER SIX

Smart Snacks for Between Meals

Nutrient-Dense Snack Ideas to Keep Blood Sugar Stable

Choosing nutrient-dense snacks can help keep blood sugar levels stable between meals while providing essential nutrients to support overall health. Here are some ideas for nutrient-dense snacks:

Greek Yogurt with Berries: Greek yogurt is rich in protein, which helps keep you feeling full and satisfied, while berries provide fiber and antioxidants. Top a serving of Greek yogurt with fresh or frozen berries like strawberries, blueberries, or raspberries for a delicious and nutritious snack.

Raw Vegetables with Hummus: Crunchy raw vegetables like carrot sticks, cucumber slices, bell pepper strips, and cherry tomatoes are low in calories and high in fiber, vitamins, and minerals. Pair them with a serving of hummus for a satisfying snack that provides protein, healthy fats, and additional flavor.

Hard-Boiled Eggs: Hard-boiled eggs are a convenient and portable snack that's packed with protein and essential nutrients like vitamin D and B vitamins. Enjoy a hard-boiled egg on its own or slice it and sprinkle with salt, pepper, and a pinch of paprika for extra flavor.

Mixed Nuts and Seeds: Nuts and seeds are rich in healthy fats, protein, and fiber, making them a satisfying and nutritious snack option. Choose unsalted varieties like almonds, walnuts, cashews, pistachios, pumpkin seeds, and sunflower seeds, and portion them out into individual servings for portion control.

Apple Slices with Almond Butter: Apple slices are a naturally sweet and crunchy snack that's high in fiber and antioxidants. Pair them with a tablespoon of almond butter or peanut butter for a delicious combination of flavors and textures that will keep you satisfied until your next meal.

Homemade Snacks That Are Low in Added Sugar and High in Flavor

Making your own snacks at home allows you to control the ingredients and ensure they're low in added sugar and high in flavor. Here are some homemade snack ideas to try:

Trail Mix: Make your own trail mix by combining unsalted nuts, seeds, and dried fruits like almonds, cashews, pumpkin seeds, sunflower seeds, raisins, dried cranberries, and apricots. Portion out individual servings into small containers or resealable bags for a convenient and satisfying snack.

Baked Kale Chips: Kale chips are a crunchy and nutritious alternative to potato chips that are easy to make at home. Tear kale leaves into bite-sized pieces, toss with olive oil, salt, and your favorite seasonings, then spread them out on a baking sheet and bake until crisp. Enjoy them on their own or with a sprinkle of Parmesan cheese for extra flavor.

Homemade Energy Balls: Energy balls are portable and easy to customize with your favorite ingredients. Combine rolled oats, nut butter, honey or maple syrup, and mix-ins like chopped nuts, seeds, dried fruits, chocolate chips, or coconut flakes. Roll the mixture into bite-sized balls and refrigerate until firm. These energy balls are perfect for a quick pick-me-up between meals.

Roasted Chickpeas: Roasted chickpeas are a crunchy and satisfying snack that's high in protein and fiber. Drain and rinse canned chickpeas, then toss them with olive oil and seasonings like garlic powder, paprika, and cumin. Spread them out on a baking sheet and bake until crispy. Enjoy them on their own or as a topping for salads and soups.

Portable Snacks for On-the-Go Convenience

When you're on the go, having portable snacks on hand can help you stay fueled and satisfied throughout the day. Here are some convenient options:

String Cheese: String cheese is a convenient and portable snack that's rich in protein and calcium. Pack individual string cheese sticks in your bag or purse for a quick and satisfying snack when you're on the go.

Whole Fruit: Fresh fruit like apples, bananas, oranges, and grapes are naturally portable and require no preparation. Pack a piece of whole fruit in your bag or backpack for a nutritious and convenient snack that's ready to eat whenever hunger strikes.

Rice Cakes with Nut Butter: Rice cakes are a crunchy and low-calorie snack that pairs well with nut butter for added protein and flavor. Spread a rice cake with almond butter, peanut butter, or sunflower seed butter for a satisfying and portable snack option.

Greek Yogurt Cups: Single-serve cups of Greek yogurt are convenient for on-the-go snacking and come in a variety of flavors and toppings. Look for options that are low in added sugars and high in protein for a nutritious and satisfying snack.

Dried Seaweed Snacks: Dried seaweed snacks are lightweight, portable, and packed with nutrients like vitamins, minerals, and antioxidants. They come in individual packets or larger sheets that can be easily broken into smaller pieces for snacking on the go.

In summary, smart snacks for between meals should be nutrient-dense, low in added sugar, and convenient for on-the-go consumption. Whether you choose pre-packaged options or make your own homemade snacks at home, aim to include a balance of protein, fiber, healthy fats, and carbohydrates to keep you fueled and satisfied throughout the day. Experiment with different flavors, textures, and combinations to find snacks that you enjoy and that support your health and well-being.

CHAPTER SEVEN

Delectable Desserts Without the Guilt

Lower-Sugar Dessert Recipes for Sweet Cravings

Satisfying your sweet tooth without consuming excessive sugar is possible with lower-sugar dessert recipes. Here are some ideas to indulge your cravings guilt-free:

Dark Chocolate Covered Almonds: Coat whole almonds in melted dark chocolate with at least 70% cocoa content. Place them on a parchment-lined tray and let them cool until the chocolate hardens. Dark chocolate contains less sugar than milk chocolate and is rich in antioxidants, making it a healthier option for a sweet treat.

Baked Apples with Cinnamon: Core apples and sprinkle them with cinnamon and a touch of honey or maple syrup. Bake until tender and fragrant. Baked apples are naturally sweet and require minimal added sugar, making them a satisfying dessert option that's perfect for chilly evenings.

Chia Seed Pudding: Mix chia seeds with unsweetened almond milk or coconut milk and a natural sweetener like stevia or monk fruit. Let the mixture sit in the refrigerator until thickened, then top with fresh fruit, nuts, or a sprinkle of cinnamon for added flavor. Chia seed pudding is high in fiber and omega-3 fatty acids, making it a nutritious and satisfying dessert.

Frozen Yogurt Bark: Spread Greek yogurt onto a parchment-lined baking sheet and top with chopped fruit, nuts, and a drizzle of honey or agave syrup. Freeze until firm, then break into pieces for a refreshing and low-sugar dessert option. Greek yogurt is high in protein and probiotics, while fruit provides natural sweetness and vitamins.

Fruit-Based Desserts That Are Naturally Sweet and Diabetic-Friendly

Fruit-based desserts are naturally sweet and full of vitamins, minerals, and fiber, making them ideal for people with diabetes. Here are some delicious options to try:

Grilled Pineapple with Cinnamon: Slice fresh pineapple into rings and grill until caramelized and slightly charred. Sprinkle with cinnamon before serving for a simple and flavorful dessert that's bursting with tropical sweetness. Pineapple is rich in vitamin C and bromelain, a digestive enzyme that aids in digestion.

Berry Compote with Greek Yogurt: Simmer mixed berries like strawberries, blueberries, and raspberries with a splash of water and a squeeze of lemon juice until thickened. Serve the warm compote over a bowl of Greek yogurt for a colorful and nutritious dessert that's rich in antioxidants and protein.

Fruit Salad with Mint: Toss together a variety of fresh fruit like melons, berries, grapes, and citrus segments with a handful of torn mint leaves. Squeeze a bit of lime juice over the fruit to enhance the flavors. Fruit salad is a refreshing and hydrating dessert option that's perfect for warm weather.

Frozen Banana "Nice" Cream: Blend frozen bananas with a splash of milk or coconut milk until smooth and creamy. Add flavorings like cocoa powder, vanilla extract, or peanut butter for extra indulgence. Frozen banana "nice" cream is naturally sweet and creamy, making it a satisfying alternative to traditional ice cream.

Indulgent Treats Made Healthier with Smart Ingredient Swaps

Enjoying indulgent treats doesn't have to derail your healthy eating goals. By making smart ingredient swaps, you can create healthier versions of your favorite desserts. Here are some ideas:

Avocado Chocolate Mousse: Blend ripe avocados with cocoa powder, a natural sweetener like honey or agave syrup, and a splash of almond milk until smooth and creamy. Avocado chocolate mousse is rich and decadent, with the added benefit of heart-healthy fats and fiber.

Oatmeal Raisin Cookies: Swap out traditional white flour for whole wheat flour or oat flour, and reduce the amount of sugar by using a combination of natural sweeteners like mashed bananas, applesauce, or dates. Add raisins, cinnamon, and a touch of vanilla extract for classic oatmeal raisin cookie flavor without the guilt.

Baked Oatmeal Bars: Mix rolled oats with mashed bananas, almond milk, and a natural sweetener like maple syrup or honey. Fold in add-ins like nuts, seeds, dried fruit, or chocolate chips, then press the mixture into a baking dish and bake until golden and set. Cut into bars for a wholesome and portable dessert or snack option.

Coconut Flour Pancakes: Substitute coconut flour for traditional wheat flour in pancake recipes to increase fiber and reduce carbohydrates. Use unsweetened applesauce or mashed bananas to add moisture and natural sweetness, and top with fresh fruit, Greek yogurt, or a drizzle of pure maple syrup for a satisfying breakfast or dessert.

In conclusion, enjoying delicious desserts without the guilt is possible with lower-sugar recipes, fruit-based options, and smart ingredient swaps. Whether you're craving something sweet and decadent or light and refreshing, there are plenty of nutritious and satisfying dessert options to choose from. Experiment with different flavors, textures, and ingredients to find desserts that satisfy your cravings while supporting your health and well-being.

CHAPTER EIGHT

Flavorful Side Dishes to Accompany Any Meal

Simple Vegetable Side Dishes Packed with Nutrients

Incorporating vegetable side dishes into your meals is a great way to add flavor, texture, and nutrition. Here are some simple and nutritious vegetable side dishes to complement any meal:

Roasted Vegetables: Toss chopped vegetables like carrots, bell peppers, zucchini, and Brussels sprouts with olive oil, salt, pepper, and your favorite herbs and spices. Roast in the oven until caramelized and tender for a flavorful and colorful side dish that pairs well with grilled meats, roasted chicken, or fish.

Sautéed Greens: Heat olive oil in a skillet and add thinly sliced greens like spinach, kale, Swiss chard, or collard greens. Sauté until wilted and tender, then season with garlic, lemon juice, and a pinch of red pepper flakes for added flavor. Sautéed greens are rich in vitamins, minerals, and antioxidants, making them a healthy and delicious side dish option.

Steamed Vegetables with Herbed Butter: Steam mixed vegetables like broccoli, cauliflower, and green beans until crisp-tender, then toss with melted butter infused with fresh herbs like thyme, rosemary, and parsley. Season with salt and pepper to taste for a simple yet flavorful side dish that complements a variety of main courses.

Vegetable Stir-Fry: Sauté diced vegetables like bell peppers, onions, carrots, and snap peas in a hot skillet with garlic, ginger, and soy sauce until crisp-tender. Add a splash of rice vinegar and sesame oil for extra flavor, then serve the stir-fry as a vibrant and nutritious side dish alongside rice, noodles, or protein of your choice.

Whole Grain and Legume-Based Side Dishes for Sustained Energy

Whole grains and legumes are nutritious and versatile ingredients that can be used to create hearty and satisfying side dishes. Here are some ideas to try:

Quinoa Pilaf: Cook quinoa in vegetable broth with diced onions, garlic, and your favorite herbs and spices until fluffy and tender. Stir in toasted nuts, dried fruit, and chopped fresh herbs like parsley or cilantro for added flavor and texture. Quinoa pilaf is a nutritious and protein-rich side dish that pairs well with grilled meats, roasted vegetables, or tofu.

Brown Rice Salad: Mix cooked brown rice with diced vegetables like cucumber, cherry tomatoes, bell peppers, and red onions. Toss with a vinaigrette made with olive oil, lemon juice, Dijon mustard, and herbs like basil or mint. Garnish with crumbled feta cheese or toasted pine nuts for extra flavor and crunch.

Lentil Salad: Combine cooked lentils with diced vegetables like celery, carrots, and bell peppers. Dress with a tangy vinaigrette made with red wine vinegar, olive oil, garlic, and Dijon mustard. Add fresh herbs like parsley, cilantro, or dill for a burst of flavor. Lentil salad is a protein-packed side dish that's perfect for picnics, barbecues, or potlucks.

Chickpea Curry: Simmer cooked chickpeas in a fragrant curry sauce made with coconut milk, tomatoes, onions, garlic, ginger, and spices like turmeric, cumin, and coriander. Serve the chickpea curry alongside basmati rice or naan bread for a hearty and flavorful side dish that's sure to please vegetarians and meat-eaters alike.

Creative Ways to Add Flavor to Your Side Dish Repertoire

Elevate your side dishes with creative flavor combinations and cooking techniques. Here are some ideas to inspire you:

Grilled Vegetable Skewers: Thread chunks of marinated vegetables like mushrooms, cherry tomatoes, squash, and red onions onto skewers and grill until charred and tender. Brush with a balsamic glaze or chimichurri sauce for extra flavor and serve as a colorful and flavorful side dish for grilled meats or seafood.

Cauliflower Mash: Steam or boil cauliflower florets until soft, then mash with a potato masher or blend in a food processor until smooth and creamy. Stir in roasted garlic, grated Parmesan cheese, and chopped fresh herbs like chives or thyme for a flavorful and low-carb alternative to mashed potatoes.

Spiced Roasted Sweet Potatoes: Toss sweet potato cubes with olive oil and spices like smoked paprika, cumin, and cinnamon before roasting in the oven until caramelized and crispy. Sprinkle with chopped cilantro or parsley and a squeeze of lime juice for a zesty and flavorful side dish that's perfect for fall and winter meals.

Miso Glazed Eggplant: Slice Japanese eggplants in half lengthwise and brush with a mixture of miso paste, soy sauce, rice vinegar, and honey or maple syrup. Roast in the oven until tender and caramelized, then garnish with sesame seeds and sliced green onions for a savory and umami-rich side dish that pairs well with Asian-inspired meals.

In summary, flavorful side dishes can elevate any meal and add variety and nutrition to your plate. Whether you prefer simple vegetable preparations, hearty whole grain and legume dishes, or creative flavor combinations and cooking techniques, there are endless possibilities to explore. Experiment with different ingredients, seasonings, and cooking methods to create side dishes that complement your main courses and satisfy your taste buds.

CHAPTER NINE

Entertaining and Special Occasion Menus

Hosting a Diabetic-Friendly Dinner Party or Gathering

Hosting a dinner party or gathering while considering the dietary needs of guests with diabetes requires careful planning and thoughtful menu choices. Here are some tips for hosting a diabetic-friendly event:

Focus on Whole Foods: Serve dishes made with whole, unprocessed ingredients like lean proteins, vegetables, fruits, whole grains, and healthy fats. Minimize the use of refined carbohydrates, added sugars, and processed foods to help keep blood sugar levels stable.

Offer Balanced Options: Provide a variety of dishes that include lean proteins, non-starchy vegetables, and healthy carbohydrates. Consider serving a protein-rich main course like grilled chicken, salmon, or tofu, along with plenty of vegetable side dishes and whole grain options like quinoa, brown rice, or whole wheat pasta.

Limit Added Sugars: Avoid dishes that are heavily sweetened or loaded with added sugars. Opt for naturally sweet ingredients like fresh fruits, dried fruits, and small amounts of natural sweeteners like honey or maple syrup when necessary. Be mindful of portion sizes and offer sugar-free or low-sugar dessert options for guests with diabetes.

Provide Plenty of Non-Alcoholic Beverage Options: Offer a variety of non-alcoholic beverage options like water, sparkling water, unsweetened iced tea, herbal tea, and sugar-free lemonade or fruit-infused water. Avoid sugary soft drinks and cocktails, and consider offering mocktail versions of popular drinks for guests who prefer not to drink alcohol.

Communicate with Guests: Prior to the event, communicate with guests about their dietary preferences and any specific dietary restrictions or food allergies they may have, including diabetes. Offer to accommodate their needs and provide them with information about the menu so they can make informed choices.

Tips for Navigating Holiday Meals and Festive Celebrations

Holiday meals and festive celebrations often revolve around food, making it challenging for people with diabetes to navigate. Here are some tips for enjoying holiday meals while managing diabetes:

Plan Ahead: Plan your holiday meals in advance and consider incorporating healthier versions of traditional dishes that are lower in carbohydrates and added sugars. Look for recipes that use whole, unprocessed ingredients and focus on flavor and nutrition.

Practice Portion Control: Pay attention to portion sizes and avoid overeating, especially high-carbohydrate and high-calorie foods like bread, potatoes, stuffing, and desserts. Use smaller plates and serving utensils to help control portion sizes and prevent overindulgence.

Choose Wisely: Be selective about the foods you choose to indulge in and prioritize nutrient-dense options like lean proteins, non-starchy vegetables, and whole grains. Fill your plate with plenty of colorful fruits and vegetables, and limit your intake of refined carbohydrates, sugary foods, and high-fat dishes.

Stay Active: Incorporate physical activity into your holiday festivities by going for a walk after meals, playing outdoor games with family and friends, or participating in holiday-themed activities like ice skating or sledding. Staying active can help lower blood sugar levels and offset the effects of indulging in holiday treats.

Monitor Blood Sugar Levels: Monitor your blood sugar levels regularly throughout the holiday season, especially before and after meals, to ensure they remain within your target range. Be prepared to make adjustments to your meal plan or medication regimen as needed to maintain optimal blood sugar control.

Special Occasion Menus That Wow Without Compromising Health

Creating special occasion menus that wow your guests while prioritizing health and nutrition is entirely possible. Here are some ideas for crafting memorable and health-conscious menus for special occasions:

Appetizers:

- Grilled Vegetable Platter with Hummus
- Caprese Skewers with Cherry Tomatoes, Fresh Mozzarella, and Basil
- Smoked Salmon and Cucumber Roll-Ups with Herbed Cream Cheese

Main Courses:

- Herb-Roasted Turkey Breast with Cranberry Orange Relish
- Grilled Lemon Garlic Shrimp Skewers

- Mushroom and Spinach Stuffed Chicken Breast with Balsamic Glaze
- Herb-Crusted Baked Salmon with Roasted Asparagus

Side Dishes:

- Quinoa and Roasted Vegetable Salad with Lemon Vinaigrette
- Garlic Mashed Cauliflower with Parmesan Cheese
- Roasted Brussels Sprouts with Balsamic Glaze and Toasted Pecans
- Wild Rice Pilaf with Dried Cranberries and Toasted Almonds

Desserts:

- Mixed Berry Parfait with Greek Yogurt and Almond Granola
- Dark Chocolate Dipped Strawberries
- Mini Fruit Tartlets with Almond Flour Crust
- Coconut Milk Panna Cotta with Fresh Berries

In conclusion, hosting a diabetic-friendly dinner party or navigating holiday meals and festive celebrations requires thoughtful planning and consideration. By focusing on whole foods, balanced options, portion control, and mindful choices, you can create memorable and health-conscious menus that wow your guests without compromising health. Experiment with flavorful ingredients, creative recipes, and nutrient-dense dishes to make every occasion special and enjoyable for everyone, including those with diabetes.

Mediterranean Diet:

Definition:

The Mediterranean diet is inspired by the traditional dietary patterns of countries bordering the Mediterranean Sea. It emphasizes whole, minimally processed foods such as fruits, vegetables, whole grains, nuts, seeds, legumes, fish, and olive oil. It limits red meat and sweets, while encouraging moderate consumption of dairy products, poultry, and eggs.

Ingredients:

- Fruits: Berries, apples, oranges, grapes, etc.
- Vegetables: Spinach, tomatoes, peppers, onions, etc.
- Whole Grains: Whole wheat bread, brown rice, quinoa, oats, etc.
- Nuts and Seeds: Almonds, walnuts, flaxseeds, chia seeds, etc.
- Legumes: Chickpeas, lentils, beans, etc.

- Fish and Seafood: Salmon, tuna, shrimp, etc.
- Olive Oil: Extra virgin olive oil for cooking and dressing.
- Herbs and Spices: Basil, oregano, garlic, cumin, etc.

Instructions/How to Prepare:

1. Base meals around plant-based foods like fruits, vegetables, whole grains, and legumes.
2. Use olive oil as the primary source of fat for cooking and dressing salads.
3. Incorporate fish and seafood into your diet regularly, aiming for at least two servings per week.
4. Enjoy moderate amounts of poultry, eggs, and dairy products, such as yogurt and cheese.
5. Limit red meat consumption to a few times per month.
6. Snack on nuts and seeds for a healthy source of fats and protein.
7. Flavor meals with herbs and spices instead of salt.
8. Drink plenty of water and enjoy a moderate amount of red wine if desired (optional).

DASH Diet (Dietary Approaches to Stop Hypertension):

Definition:

The DASH diet is specifically designed to help lower blood pressure and reduce the risk of hypertension. It emphasizes fruits, vegetables, whole grains, and lean proteins while limiting sodium, saturated fats, and sweets.

Ingredients:

- Fruits: Berries, bananas, apples, oranges, etc.
- Vegetables: Leafy greens, carrots, broccoli, bell peppers, etc.
- Whole Grains: Brown rice, whole wheat bread, quinoa, oats, barley, etc.
- Lean Proteins: Chicken breast, turkey, fish, tofu, beans, lentils, etc.
- Dairy: Low-fat or fat-free milk, yogurt, cheese, etc.
- Nuts and Seeds: Almonds, pistachios, sunflower seeds, etc.
- Healthy Fats: Olive oil, avocado, nuts, seeds, etc.

Instructions/How to Prepare:

1. Focus on incorporating plenty of fruits and vegetables into your meals and snacks.
2. Choose whole grains over refined grains whenever possible.
3. Opt for lean proteins such as poultry, fish, tofu, and legumes.

4. Limit high-fat dairy products and opt for low-fat or fat-free options.

5. Include nuts and seeds as snacks or in salads for added nutrients and healthy fats.

6. Use herbs, spices, and citrus juices to flavor foods instead of salt.

7. Avoid processed and high-sodium foods like canned soups, packaged snacks, and fast food.

8. Cook meals at home whenever possible to have better control over ingredients and portion sizes.

9. Aim to limit sweets and sugary beverages, opting for natural sweeteners like fruit when craving something sweet.

10. Stay hydrated by drinking plenty of water throughout the day.

Low-Carb Diet:

Definition:

A low-carb diet involves reducing carbohydrate intake while increasing the consumption of protein and healthy fats. This diet aims to control insulin levels, promote weight loss, and improve overall health by limiting foods high in carbohydrates such as bread, pasta, rice, and sugary snacks.

Ingredients:

- Protein Sources: Meat, poultry, fish, tofu, tempeh, eggs.
- Non-Starchy Vegetables: Leafy greens, broccoli, cauliflower, zucchini, bell peppers.
- Healthy Fats: Avocado, nuts, seeds, olive oil, coconut oil.
- Dairy: Cheese, Greek yogurt, cottage cheese (in moderation).
- Low-Carb Fruits: Berries, avocados, tomatoes, lemons, limes.
- Herbs and Spices: Basil, oregano, garlic, turmeric, cumin.
- Sweeteners (optional): Stevia, erythritol, monk fruit.

Instructions/How to Prepare:

1. Focus on whole, unprocessed foods.
2. Limit carbohydrate intake to around 20-50 grams per day, depending on individual needs and goals.
3. Include protein-rich foods in each meal to promote satiety and muscle maintenance.
4. Fill up on non-starchy vegetables to increase fiber intake and provide essential vitamins and minerals.
5. Incorporate healthy fats into your diet for energy and to keep you feeling full.

6. Be mindful of hidden carbs in sauces, condiments, and processed foods.

7. Drink plenty of water to stay hydrated and support overall health.

8. Experiment with low-carb recipes and meal prep to make adhering to the diet easier and more enjoyable.

Ketogenic Diet (Keto Diet):

Definition:

The ketogenic diet is a very low-carb, high-fat diet that forces the body to enter a state of ketosis, where it primarily burns fat for fuel instead of carbohydrates. This diet has been used for decades to treat epilepsy and has gained popularity for weight loss and improving metabolic health.

Ingredients:

- Healthy Fats: Avocado, coconut oil, olive oil, butter, ghee, fatty fish.

- Protein Sources: Meat, poultry, fish, eggs, tofu, tempeh.

- Non-Starchy Vegetables: Leafy greens, broccoli, cauliflower, zucchini, asparagus.

- Full-Fat Dairy: Cheese, heavy cream, Greek yogurt (in moderation).

- Nuts and Seeds: Macadamia nuts, almonds, chia seeds, flaxseeds.

- Low-Carb Fruits: Berries (in moderation), avocado.

- Herbs and Spices: Turmeric, ginger, cinnamon, garlic, thyme.

- Sweeteners (in moderation): Stevia, erythritol, monk fruit.

Instructions/How to Prepare:

1. Keep carbohydrate intake extremely low, typically below 20-50 grams per day to induce and maintain ketosis.

2. Consume moderate amounts of protein, as excessive protein intake can potentially hinder ketosis.

3. Base meals around healthy fats, such as avocados, olive oil, and fatty fish.

4. Incorporate non-starchy vegetables to provide essential nutrients and fiber while keeping carbohydrate intake low.

5. Be mindful of hidden carbs in foods and beverages, including sauces, dressings, and flavored beverages.

6. Stay hydrated by drinking plenty of water, as dehydration can occur more easily on a ketogenic diet.

7. Monitor ketone levels using urine strips, blood tests, or breath meters if desired, to ensure you are in ketosis.

8. Experiment with keto-friendly recipes and meal planning to maintain variety and enjoyment while following the diet.

Plant-Based Diet:

Definition:

A plant-based diet primarily consists of foods derived from plants, such as fruits, vegetables, grains, nuts, seeds, and legumes. It emphasizes whole, minimally processed foods while minimizing or eliminating animal products. The focus is on incorporating a variety of plant foods to promote health and well-being.

Ingredients:

- Fruits: Berries, apples, oranges, bananas, etc.
- Vegetables: Leafy greens, broccoli, carrots, bell peppers, etc.
- Whole Grains: Brown rice, quinoa, oats, barley, whole wheat bread, etc.
- Legumes: Chickpeas, lentils, black beans, kidney beans, etc.
- Nuts and Seeds: Almonds, walnuts, chia seeds, flaxseeds, pumpkin seeds, etc.
- Plant-Based Proteins: Tofu, tempeh, seitan, edamame, plant-based protein powders, etc.
- Healthy Fats: Avocado, olive oil, coconut oil, nuts, seeds, etc.

Instructions/How to Prepare:

1. Base meals around a variety of whole plant foods, including fruits, vegetables, whole grains, legumes, nuts, and seeds.

2. Incorporate a rainbow of colorful fruits and vegetables to ensure a diverse array of nutrients.

3. Include plant-based proteins such as tofu, tempeh, and legumes in meals to meet protein needs.

4. Choose whole grains over refined grains for added fiber and nutrients.

5. Experiment with different cooking methods, such as steaming, roasting, sautéing, and grilling, to enhance flavor and texture.

6. Use herbs, spices, and condiments to add flavor to dishes without relying on animal products.

7. Be mindful of nutrient needs, particularly vitamin B12, vitamin D, omega-3 fatty acids, iron, calcium, and zinc, and consider supplementation if necessary.

8. Stay hydrated by drinking plenty of water throughout the day.

9. Plan balanced meals and snacks to ensure adequate intake of essential nutrients.

10. Enjoy plant-based alternatives to dairy and meat products, such as plant-based milk, cheese, yogurt, and meat substitutes, if desired.

Vegan Diet:

Definition:

A vegan diet excludes all animal products, including meat, poultry, fish, dairy, eggs, and honey. It is based entirely on plant foods and emphasizes cruelty-free living and environmental sustainability.

Ingredients:

- Fruits: Berries, apples, oranges, mangoes, etc.
- Vegetables: Spinach, kale, tomatoes, onions, mushrooms, etc.
- Whole Grains: Quinoa, brown rice, barley, whole wheat pasta, etc.
- Legumes: Chickpeas, black beans, lentils, kidney beans, etc.
- Nuts and Seeds: Almonds, cashews, sunflower seeds, chia seeds, etc.
- Plant-Based Proteins: Tofu, tempeh, seitan, soy-based meat substitutes, etc.
- Healthy Fats: Avocado, olive oil, coconut oil, nuts, seeds, etc.

- Plant-Based Dairy Alternatives: Almond milk, coconut milk, soy milk, vegan cheese, vegan yogurt, etc.

Instructions/How to Prepare:

1. Build meals around plant foods, including fruits, vegetables, whole grains, legumes, nuts, and seeds.

2. Ensure adequate protein intake by including sources such as tofu, tempeh, legumes, and plant-based meat substitutes.

3. Use plant-based milk, cheese, and yogurt alternatives in place of dairy products.

4. Experiment with vegan cooking techniques and recipes to discover new flavors and textures.

5. Pay attention to nutrient needs, especially vitamin B12, vitamin D, omega-3 fatty acids, iron, calcium, and zinc, and consider supplementation if necessary.

6. Read labels carefully to avoid hidden animal ingredients in processed foods and beverages.

7. Be mindful of cross-contamination when preparing and consuming food to prevent unintentional consumption of animal products.

8. Explore vegan-friendly restaurants and eateries or plan ahead when dining out to ensure vegan options are available.

9. Connect with vegan communities and resources for support, recipe ideas, and lifestyle tips.

10. Embrace the ethical and environmental principles of veganism beyond diet by choosing cruelty-free and sustainable products in other areas of life, such as clothing, cosmetics, and household items.

Vegetarian Diet:

Definition:

A vegetarian diet excludes meat, poultry, and seafood, but includes plant-based foods such as fruits, vegetables, grains, nuts, seeds, and dairy products. There are different variations of vegetarianism, including lacto-vegetarian (includes dairy but not eggs), ovo-vegetarian (includes eggs but not dairy), and lacto-ovo-vegetarian (includes both dairy and eggs).

Ingredients:

- Fruits: Berries, apples, oranges, bananas, etc.
- Vegetables: Leafy greens, broccoli, carrots, bell peppers, etc.
- Whole Grains: Brown rice, quinoa, oats, barley, whole wheat bread, etc.
- Legumes: Chickpeas, lentils, black beans, kidney beans, etc.

- Nuts and Seeds: Almonds, walnuts, chia seeds, flaxseeds, pumpkin seeds, etc.

- Dairy: Milk, yogurt, cheese, butter, etc. (depending on the type of vegetarianism)

- Plant-Based Proteins: Tofu, tempeh, seitan, edamame, etc.

- Healthy Fats: Avocado, olive oil, coconut oil, nuts, seeds, etc.

Instructions/How to Prepare:

1. Base meals around a variety of plant foods, including fruits, vegetables, whole grains, legumes, nuts, and seeds.

2. Incorporate plant-based proteins such as tofu, tempeh, legumes, nuts, and seeds into meals to meet protein needs.

3. Choose whole grains over refined grains for added fiber and nutrients.

4. Experiment with different cooking methods, such as steaming, roasting, sautéing, and grilling, to enhance flavor and texture.

5. Use herbs, spices, and condiments to add flavor to dishes without relying on meat.

6. Be mindful of nutrient needs, especially vitamin B12, vitamin D, omega-3 fatty acids, iron, calcium, and zinc, and consider supplementation if necessary.

7. Stay hydrated by drinking plenty of water throughout the day.

8. Plan balanced meals and snacks to ensure adequate intake of essential nutrients.

9. Explore vegetarian cooking techniques and recipes to discover new flavors and textures.

10. Connect with vegetarian communities and resources for support, recipe ideas, and lifestyle tips.

Atkins Diet:

Definition:

The Atkins diet is a low-carbohydrate, high-fat diet designed for weight loss and improving overall health. It involves reducing carbohydrate intake while increasing the consumption of protein and healthy fats. The diet is divided into four phases: induction, balancing, fine-tuning, and maintenance.

Ingredients:

- Protein Sources: Meat, poultry, fish, eggs, tofu, tempeh, etc.
- Non-Starchy Vegetables: Leafy greens, broccoli, cauliflower, zucchini, bell peppers, etc.
- Healthy Fats: Avocado, olive oil, coconut oil, butter, ghee, fatty fish, etc.

- Full-Fat Dairy (in moderation): Cheese, Greek yogurt, heavy cream, etc.

- Nuts and Seeds (in moderation): Almonds, walnuts, chia seeds, flaxseeds, etc.

- Low-Carb Fruits (in moderation): Berries, avocados, tomatoes, etc.

- Herbs and Spices: Basil, oregano, garlic, turmeric, cumin, etc.

Instructions/How to Prepare:

1. Start with the induction phase, which restricts carbohydrate intake to 20-25 grams per day for two weeks to induce ketosis.

2. Base meals around protein-rich foods such as meat, poultry, fish, eggs, and tofu.

3. Include non-starchy vegetables to provide essential nutrients and fiber while keeping carbohydrate intake low.

4. Incorporate healthy fats into your diet for energy and to keep you feeling full.

5. Gradually increase carbohydrate intake during the balancing, fine-tuning, and maintenance phases while monitoring weight and overall health.

6. Be mindful of portion sizes and track carbohydrate intake to stay within the recommended limits for each phase.

7. Stay hydrated by drinking plenty of water throughout the day.

8. Experiment with low-carb recipes and meal planning to maintain variety and enjoyment while following the diet.

9. Consider working with a healthcare professional or registered dietitian to personalize the diet plan and ensure nutritional adequacy.

10. Monitor progress and make adjustments as needed to achieve weight loss and health goals.

South Beach Diet:

Definition:

The South Beach Diet is a popular weight-loss program that emphasizes the consumption of lean protein, healthy fats, and low-glycemic carbohydrates. It's divided into three phases: Phase 1, which eliminates most carbs to jump-start weight loss; Phase 2, which reintroduces some carbs while continuing weight loss; and Phase 3, which focuses on maintaining weight loss with a balanced diet.

Ingredients:

- Lean Proteins: Chicken breast, turkey, fish, seafood, lean cuts of beef and pork.

- Healthy Fats: Olive oil, avocado, nuts, seeds, fatty fish like salmon and mackerel.

- Low-Glycemic Carbohydrates: Non-starchy vegetables (e.g., spinach, broccoli, cauliflower), whole grains (e.g., quinoa, barley), legumes (e.g., beans, lentils).

- Low-Fat Dairy: Greek yogurt, skim milk, low-fat cheese.

Instructions/How to Prepare:

1. Phase 1: Eliminate most carbohydrates, including fruits, grains, and starchy vegetables. Focus on lean proteins, non-starchy vegetables, and healthy fats. Drink plenty of water and avoid processed foods and added sugars.

2. Phase 2: Gradually reintroduce some carbohydrates, such as fruits and whole grains, while continuing to prioritize lean proteins and healthy fats. Monitor portion sizes and continue to avoid refined sugars and processed foods.

3. Phase 3: Transition to a balanced diet that includes a variety of foods from all food groups. Focus on portion control, mindful eating, and regular physical activity to maintain weight loss and overall health.

Paleo Diet:

Definition:

The Paleo diet, also known as the Paleolithic or caveman diet, is based on the presumed diet of ancient humans during the Paleolithic era. It emphasizes whole foods that would have been available to our hunter-gatherer ancestors, such as lean meats, fish, fruits, vegetables, nuts, and seeds, while excluding processed foods, grains, legumes, and dairy products.

Ingredients:

- Lean Meats: Beef, chicken, turkey, pork, lamb, etc.
- Fish and Seafood: Salmon, trout, shrimp, shellfish, etc.
- Fruits: Berries, apples, oranges, bananas, etc.
- Vegetables: Leafy greens, broccoli, carrots, peppers, onions, etc.
- Nuts and Seeds: Almonds, walnuts, cashews, sunflower seeds, etc.
- Healthy Fats: Avocado, olive oil, coconut oil, ghee.
- Herbs and Spices: Basil, oregano, garlic, turmeric, cinnamon, etc.

Instructions/How to Prepare:

1. Base meals around lean proteins, including meat, fish, and seafood.

2. Incorporate a variety of colorful fruits and vegetables for essential vitamins, minerals, and fiber.

3. Include nuts and seeds as snacks or to add texture and flavor to meals.

4. Use healthy fats like olive oil, avocado, and coconut oil for cooking and dressing.

5. Avoid processed foods, grains, legumes, dairy products, refined sugars, and artificial additives.

6. Experiment with cooking methods such as grilling, baking, and sautéing to enhance flavor and texture.

7. Stay hydrated by drinking plenty of water throughout the day.

8. Listen to your body's hunger and fullness cues and eat mindfully.

9. Be aware of portion sizes and adjust based on individual energy needs and activity levels.

10. Focus on whole, nutrient-dense foods and prioritize quality over quantity.

Whole30 Diet:

Definition:

The Whole30 diet is a 30-day elimination diet designed to reset your body and identify potential food sensitivities. It involves removing certain food groups known to cause inflammation and digestive issues, such as sugar, grains, dairy, legumes, and processed foods, for 30 days. After the elimination period, foods are gradually reintroduced to identify which ones may be causing adverse reactions.

Ingredients:

- Protein Sources: Meat, poultry, fish, seafood, eggs.
- Vegetables: Leafy greens, cruciferous vegetables, peppers, squash, etc.
- Fruits: Berries, apples, oranges, bananas, etc.
- Healthy Fats: Avocado, olive oil, coconut oil, nuts, seeds.
- Herbs and Spices: Basil, oregano, garlic, turmeric, cinnamon, etc.

Instructions/How to Prepare:

1. Eliminate sugar, grains, dairy, legumes, and processed foods from your diet for 30 days.
2. Base meals around protein sources, including meat, poultry, fish, seafood, and eggs.

3. Include a variety of vegetables for essential vitamins, minerals, and fiber.
4. Incorporate fruits as snacks or to add natural sweetness to meals.
5. Use healthy fats like avocado, olive oil, and coconut oil for cooking and dressing.
6. Experiment with herbs and spices to enhance flavor without added sugars or artificial additives.
7. Be mindful of hidden sources of sugar and processed ingredients in condiments and packaged foods.
8. Read labels carefully and opt for whole, minimally processed foods.
9. Stay hydrated by drinking plenty of water throughout the day.
10. After the 30-day elimination period, reintroduce eliminated foods one at a time and monitor for any adverse reactions or changes in symptoms.

Low-Glycemic Index Diet:

Definition:

The Low-Glycemic Index (GI) diet focuses on consuming foods that have a low glycemic index, which means they cause a slower and more gradual increase in blood sugar levels. This diet can help stabilize blood sugar, improve insulin sensitivity, and promote weight loss. Foods with a low GI typically include non-starchy vegetables, whole grains, lean proteins, and healthy fats.

Ingredients:

- Non-Starchy Vegetables: Leafy greens, broccoli, cauliflower, peppers, carrots, etc.

- Whole Grains: Quinoa, barley, bulgur, oats, brown rice, etc.

- Lean Proteins: Chicken breast, turkey, fish, tofu, tempeh, beans, lentils.

- Healthy Fats: Avocado, olive oil, nuts, seeds, fatty fish like salmon.

- Low-Glycemic Fruits (in moderation): Berries, apples, oranges, pears, etc.

- Herbs and Spices: Basil, oregano, garlic, turmeric, cinnamon, etc.

Instructions/How to Prepare:

1. Choose whole, minimally processed foods with a low glycemic index.

2. Base meals around non-starchy vegetables, whole grains, and lean proteins.

3. Incorporate healthy fats like avocado, olive oil, nuts, and seeds for satiety and flavor.
4. Limit high-glycemic foods such as refined grains, sugary snacks, and sweetened beverages.
5. Include low-glycemic fruits in moderation, focusing on berries, apples, and citrus fruits.
6. Be mindful of portion sizes and avoid overeating, even with low-GI foods.
7. Experiment with cooking methods such as steaming, roasting, and sautéing to enhance flavor and texture.
8. Eat balanced meals that combine protein, carbohydrates, and healthy fats to promote satiety and stabilize blood sugar levels.
9. Monitor blood sugar levels if necessary and adjust your diet accordingly.
10. Stay hydrated by drinking plenty of water throughout the day.

Low-Fat Diet:

Definition:

A low-fat diet is characterized by reducing the intake of dietary fats, particularly saturated fats and trans fats, to promote heart health, manage weight, and reduce the risk of certain chronic diseases such as cardiovascular disease. This diet typically involves limiting foods high in fat and choosing lean protein sources, whole grains, fruits, vegetables, and low-fat dairy products.

Ingredients:

- Lean Proteins: Skinless poultry, lean cuts of beef and pork, fish, tofu, tempeh, legumes.

- Whole Grains: Brown rice, quinoa, barley, whole wheat bread, oats, whole grain pasta.

- Fruits: Berries, apples, oranges, bananas, grapes, etc.

- Vegetables: Leafy greens, broccoli, carrots, bell peppers, tomatoes, etc.

- Low-Fat or Fat-Free Dairy: Skim milk, low-fat yogurt, reduced-fat cheese.

- Healthy Fats (in moderation): Avocado, nuts, seeds, olive oil.

Instructions/How to Prepare:

1. Choose lean protein sources such as poultry, fish, tofu, and legumes instead of high-fat meats.

2. Opt for whole grains like brown rice, quinoa, and whole wheat bread over refined grains.

3. Include a variety of fruits and vegetables in your meals and snacks for added vitamins, minerals, and fiber.

4. Select low-fat or fat-free dairy products to reduce saturated fat intake.

5. Limit added fats and oils, and use healthier cooking methods such as baking, grilling, steaming, or boiling.

6. Be mindful of portion sizes to avoid overconsumption of calories, even with low-fat foods.

7. Read food labels to identify hidden sources of fat and choose lower-fat options when available.

8. Incorporate healthy fats like avocado, nuts, and olive oil in moderation for flavor and satiety.

9. Stay hydrated by drinking plenty of water throughout the day.

10. Focus on overall dietary patterns rather than just reducing fat intake, and aim for a balanced diet that includes a variety of nutrient-dense foods.

High-Fiber Diet:

Definition:

A high-fiber diet focuses on increasing the intake of dietary fiber, which offers numerous health benefits such as improving digestion, promoting satiety, stabilizing blood sugar levels, and reducing the risk of chronic diseases such as heart disease, diabetes, and certain cancers. This diet emphasizes whole, unprocessed foods rich in fiber, including fruits, vegetables, whole grains, legumes, nuts, and seeds.

Ingredients:

- Whole Grains: Oats, barley, quinoa, brown rice, whole wheat bread, whole grain pasta.

- Fruits: Berries, apples, oranges, pears, bananas, avocados, etc.

- Vegetables: Leafy greens, broccoli, carrots, Brussels sprouts, sweet potatoes, etc.

- Legumes: Lentils, chickpeas, black beans, kidney beans, peas, etc.

- Nuts and Seeds: Almonds, chia seeds, flaxseeds, pumpkin seeds, sunflower seeds, etc.

- Healthy Fats: Avocado, nuts, seeds, olive oil, flaxseed oil.

Instructions/How to Prepare:

1. Incorporate a variety of whole grains, fruits, vegetables, legumes, nuts, and seeds into your meals and snacks.

2. Choose whole fruits and vegetables over fruit juices and refined grains to maximize fiber intake.

3. Include high-fiber foods such as beans, lentils, and chickpeas in soups, salads, and main dishes.

4. Replace refined grains with whole grains in recipes and meals, such as swapping white rice for brown rice or white bread for whole wheat bread.

5. Snack on raw vegetables with hummus or nut butter for a fiber-rich snack.

6. Add nuts, seeds, and avocado to salads, yogurt, or smoothies for added fiber and healthy fats.

7. Be sure to drink plenty of water throughout the day to help move fiber through the digestive tract and prevent constipation.

8. Gradually increase fiber intake to allow your digestive system to adjust and minimize discomfort.

9. Monitor portion sizes, especially with high-calorie fiber-rich foods like nuts and seeds.

10. Aim to include a variety of fiber sources in your diet to ensure you're getting a balance of soluble and insoluble fiber, which offer different health benefits.

Flexitarian Diet:

Definition:

The Flexitarian diet is a flexible approach to eating that emphasizes plant-based foods while allowing for occasional consumption of meat and other animal products. It encourages individuals to primarily eat fruits, vegetables, whole grains, legumes, nuts, and seeds, while minimizing intake of processed foods, sugar, and refined grains. The diet is flexible and adaptable, making it suitable for various lifestyles and preferences.

Ingredients:

- Plant-Based Foods: Fruits, vegetables, whole grains, legumes, nuts, seeds.

- Lean Proteins: Tofu, tempeh, beans, lentils, chickpeas, edamame.

- Healthy Fats: Avocado, nuts, seeds, olive oil.

- Dairy and Eggs (optional): Greek yogurt, eggs, low-fat cheese.

- Occasional Meat and Fish: Lean cuts of poultry, fish, seafood (optional).

Instructions/How to Prepare:

1. Base meals around plant-based foods such as fruits, vegetables, whole grains, legumes, nuts, and seeds.

2. Include a variety of colorful fruits and vegetables to ensure a diverse intake of nutrients.

3. Incorporate plant-based proteins like tofu, tempeh, beans, and lentils into meals and snacks.

4. Choose healthy fats like avocado, nuts, seeds, and olive oil for cooking and dressing.

5. Limit consumption of processed foods, refined grains, and added sugars.

6. Enjoy occasional servings of lean meats, poultry, or fish if desired, but prioritize plant-based meals.

7. Be mindful of portion sizes and listen to your body's hunger and fullness cues.

8. Experiment with plant-based cooking techniques and recipes to discover new flavors and textures.

9. Stay hydrated by drinking plenty of water throughout the day.

10. Focus on long-term sustainability and balance rather than strict adherence to rules, allowing for flexibility and enjoyment in your eating habits.

Ornish Diet:

Definition:

The Ornish diet, developed by Dr. Dean Ornish, is a low-fat, plant-based eating plan designed to prevent and reverse heart disease and promote overall health and well-being. It emphasizes whole, unprocessed foods such as fruits, vegetables, whole grains, legumes, and limited amounts of low-fat dairy and plant-based proteins. The diet also encourages regular exercise, stress management, and social support as part of a holistic approach to health.

Ingredients:

- Plant-Based Foods: Fruits, vegetables, whole grains, legumes, nuts, seeds.
- Low-Fat Dairy: Skim milk, low-fat yogurt, cottage cheese (in moderation).
- Lean Proteins: Tofu, tempeh, beans, lentils, chickpeas, edamame.
- Healthy Fats (in moderation): Avocado, nuts, seeds, olive oil.
- Occasional Fish (optional): Fatty fish like salmon, trout, sardines (in moderation).

Instructions/How to Prepare:

1. Base meals around plant-based foods such as fruits, vegetables, whole grains, legumes, nuts, and seeds.

2. Include a variety of colorful fruits and vegetables to ensure a diverse intake of nutrients.

3. Choose low-fat dairy products like skim milk, low-fat yogurt, and cottage cheese in moderation.

4. Incorporate plant-based proteins like tofu, tempeh, beans, and lentils into meals and snacks.

5. Limit consumption of added fats and oils, opting for healthier sources like avocado, nuts, seeds, and olive oil.

6. Minimize intake of animal products, particularly high-fat meats and full-fat dairy.

7. Focus on whole, unprocessed foods and avoid processed and refined foods.

8. Practice stress management techniques such as meditation, yoga, or deep breathing exercises.

9. Engage in regular physical activity, aiming for at least 30 minutes of moderate exercise most days of the week.

10. Cultivate a supportive social network and prioritize meaningful connections with friends and loved ones for overall well-being.

TLC Diet (Therapeutic Lifestyle Changes):

Definition:

The TLC diet is a heart-healthy eating plan designed to reduce cholesterol levels and lower the risk of heart disease. It emphasizes reducing intake of saturated fat and dietary cholesterol while focusing on consuming a variety of nutrient-rich foods, including fruits, vegetables, whole grains, lean proteins, and healthy fats. The diet also encourages regular physical activity and other lifestyle modifications to promote heart health.

Ingredients:

- Fruits: Berries, apples, oranges, bananas, grapes, etc.
- Vegetables: Leafy greens, broccoli, carrots, bell peppers, tomatoes, etc.
- Whole Grains: Oats, barley, quinoa, brown rice, whole wheat bread, whole grain pasta.
- Lean Proteins: Skinless poultry, fish, seafood, tofu, beans, lentils.
- Healthy Fats: Avocado, nuts, seeds, olive oil, fatty fish like salmon.

- Low-Fat or Fat-Free Dairy: Skim milk, low-fat yogurt, reduced-fat cheese.
- Herbs and Spices: Basil, oregano, garlic, turmeric, cinnamon, etc.

Instructions/How to Prepare:

1. Limit intake of saturated fats, trans fats, and dietary cholesterol by choosing lean proteins, low-fat dairy products, and healthy fats.
2. Focus on consuming a variety of colorful fruits and vegetables for essential vitamins, minerals, and antioxidants.
3. Choose whole grains over refined grains for added fiber and nutrients.
4. Incorporate lean proteins such as poultry, fish, tofu, beans, and lentils into meals and snacks.
5. Use healthy fats like avocado, nuts, seeds, and olive oil for cooking and dressing.
6. Limit consumption of processed foods, sugary snacks, and high-fat meats.
7. Be mindful of portion sizes to avoid overeating, especially with calorie-dense foods.

8. Read food labels to identify hidden sources of saturated and trans fats, sodium, and added sugars.

9. Stay hydrated by drinking plenty of water throughout the day.

10. Engage in regular physical activity, aiming for at least 30 minutes of moderate exercise most days of the week to complement dietary changes and promote overall heart health.

FODMAP Diet (Fermentable Oligosaccharides, Disaccharides, Monosaccharides, and Polyols):

Definition:

The FODMAP diet is a therapeutic approach to managing symptoms of irritable bowel syndrome (IBS) and other gastrointestinal disorders. It involves temporarily reducing or eliminating certain types of carbohydrates that are poorly absorbed in the small intestine and can ferment in the colon, leading to gas, bloating, abdominal pain, and other digestive symptoms. The diet consists of three phases: elimination, reintroduction, and personalization.

Ingredients:

- Low-FODMAP Fruits: Berries, citrus fruits, bananas, grapes, kiwi, etc.

- Low-FODMAP Vegetables: Leafy greens, carrots, bell peppers, zucchini, potatoes, etc.

- Low-FODMAP Grains: Quinoa, rice (white and brown), oats (gluten-free), etc.

- Low-FODMAP Proteins: Chicken, turkey, fish, eggs, tofu, tempeh, firm tofu, etc.

- Low-FODMAP Dairy: Lactose-free milk, lactose-free yogurt, hard cheeses (e.g., cheddar), etc.

- Low-FODMAP Fats and Oils: Olive oil, coconut oil, butter (in moderation), etc.

- Herbs and Spices: Basil, oregano, ginger, turmeric, cinnamon, etc.

Instructions/How to Prepare:

1. Start with the elimination phase, during which high-FODMAP foods are eliminated from the diet for 2-6 weeks to reduce symptoms.

2. Base meals around low-FODMAP foods such as fruits, vegetables, grains, proteins, and fats that are well-tolerated.

3. Gradually reintroduce high-FODMAP foods one at a time in small portions to identify trigger foods and tolerance levels.

4. Keep a food and symptom diary to track reactions to specific foods and help identify patterns.

5. Personalize the diet by incorporating a variety of low-FODMAP foods that are well-tolerated and avoiding or limiting high-FODMAP foods that trigger symptoms.

6. Be mindful of portion sizes and avoid overeating, as consuming large quantities of even low-FODMAP foods can exacerbate symptoms.

7. Consider working with a registered dietitian experienced in the FODMAP diet to ensure proper implementation and guidance throughout the process.

8. Stay hydrated by drinking plenty of water throughout the day to support digestive health.

9. Experiment with cooking methods and recipes to add flavor and variety to meals while adhering to the low-FODMAP guidelines.

10. Monitor symptoms regularly and adjust your diet as needed to manage symptoms effectively and improve overall quality of life.

Pescatarian Diet:

Definition:

The pescatarian diet is a plant-based eating pattern that includes fish and seafood but excludes other animal meats such as poultry, beef, and pork. It's a flexible approach to eating that emphasizes plant foods such as fruits, vegetables, whole grains, legumes, nuts, and seeds, while also incorporating fish and seafood for protein and essential nutrients like omega-3 fatty acids.

Ingredients:

- Fish and Seafood: Salmon, trout, tuna, mackerel, shrimp, scallops, etc.

- Plant-Based Foods: Fruits, vegetables, whole grains, legumes, nuts, seeds.

- Dairy and Eggs: Milk, cheese, yogurt, eggs (optional, depending on individual preferences).

- Healthy Fats: Avocado, olive oil, nuts, seeds.

- Herbs and Spices: Basil, oregano, garlic, turmeric, ginger, etc.

Instructions/How to Prepare:

1. Base meals around plant-based foods such as fruits, vegetables, whole grains, legumes, nuts, and seeds.

2. Incorporate fish and seafood into meals as the primary source of protein.

3. Choose fatty fish like salmon, mackerel, and trout for their omega-3 fatty acids.

4. Include dairy products and eggs if desired and tolerated, as they provide additional protein and nutrients.

5. Use healthy fats like avocado, olive oil, nuts, and seeds for cooking and dressing.

6. Experiment with a variety of cooking methods, such as grilling, baking, steaming, and sautéing, to enhance flavor and texture.

7. Be mindful of portion sizes and aim for balanced meals that include a variety of food groups.

8. Opt for whole, minimally processed foods and limit intake of processed and refined foods.

9. Stay hydrated by drinking plenty of water throughout the day.

10. Consider supplementing with vitamin B12 and vitamin D if fish and seafood are the primary sources of these nutrients in the diet.

CHAPTER TEN

Meal Planning and Prepping for Success

Strategies for Efficient Meal Planning and Grocery Shopping

Efficient meal planning and grocery shopping are essential for maintaining a healthy and balanced diet while saving time and money. Here are some strategies to help you streamline the process:

Set Aside Time for Planning: Dedicate a specific day each week to meal planning and grocery shopping. Use this time to review your schedule, inventory your pantry and fridge, and decide on meals for the upcoming week. Consider factors like dietary preferences, nutritional needs, and any special occasions or events.

Create a Weekly Meal Plan: Plan out your meals for the week, including breakfast, lunch, dinner, and snacks. Aim for a variety of nutrient-dense foods from all food groups, including fruits, vegetables, whole grains, lean proteins, and healthy fats. Write down your meal plan and post it somewhere visible, like on the fridge or a bulletin board, to help you stay organized and on track.

Make a Shopping List: Based on your meal plan, create a detailed shopping list of all the ingredients you'll need for the week. Organize your list by food categories and sections of the grocery store to make shopping more efficient. Check your pantry and fridge for items you already have on hand to avoid unnecessary purchases and food waste.

Shop with Purpose: When you go grocery shopping, stick to your list and avoid impulse purchases. Choose fresh, seasonal produce, lean proteins, whole grains, and minimally processed foods whenever possible. Compare prices, check for sales and discounts, and consider buying in bulk for items you use frequently.

Batch Cooking and Freezing Meals for Convenience

Batch cooking and freezing meals in advance can save you time and effort during busy weekdays and ensure you always have healthy options on hand. Here's how to incorporate batch cooking into your routine:

Choose Batch-Friendly Recipes: Look for recipes that are easy to scale up and freeze well, like soups, stews, casseroles, and one-pot meals. Focus on dishes that are nutrient-dense, balanced, and packed with flavor to keep you satisfied throughout the week.

Set Aside Time for Batch Cooking: Dedicate a few hours each week to batch cooking and meal prep. Choose a day when you have some free time, like a weekend or a quiet evening, and use this time to cook large batches of your favorite recipes. Divide the prepared meals into individual portions and store them in airtight containers or freezer bags for easy access.

Label and Date Everything: To avoid confusion and waste, label each container or bag with the name of the dish and the date it was prepared. This will help you keep track of what's in your freezer and how long it's been there. Use freezer-safe labels or permanent markers to ensure the labels don't smudge or fade over time.

Rotate Your Stock: Make sure to rotate your frozen meals regularly to ensure they stay fresh and don't get lost in the back of the freezer. Use a first-in, first-out (FIFO) system to prioritize older items and prevent them from becoming freezer burnt or spoiled. Keep a running inventory of your freezer contents to help you plan meals and avoid overbuying.

Tips for Maintaining a Balanced Diet and Managing Portions

Maintaining a balanced diet and managing portions is key to achieving and sustaining good health. Here are some tips to help you stay on track:

Practice Mindful Eating: Pay attention to your hunger and fullness cues, and eat slowly and attentively to fully enjoy your meals. Avoid distractions like screens or multitasking while eating, and savor the flavors, textures, and aromas of your food.

Fill Half Your Plate with Vegetables: Aim to fill at least half of your plate with non-starchy vegetables like leafy greens, broccoli, peppers, and carrots. Vegetables are low in calories and high in fiber, vitamins, and minerals, making them an essential component of a balanced diet.

Choose Whole Grains: Opt for whole grains like brown rice, quinoa, barley, oats, and whole wheat pasta over refined grains whenever possible. Whole grains are rich in fiber, which helps keep you feeling full and satisfied, and they provide essential nutrients like vitamins, minerals, and antioxidants.

Watch Portion Sizes: Be mindful of portion sizes and avoid oversized servings, especially of calorie-dense foods like pasta, rice, and high-fat dishes. Use smaller plates and bowls to help control portion sizes, and pay attention to serving sizes listed on food labels to avoid overeating.

Include Protein at Every Meal: Incorporate lean proteins like poultry, fish, tofu, beans, lentils, and Greek yogurt into your meals to help build and repair tissues, regulate hormones, and support muscle health. Aim for a palm-sized portion of protein at each meal to meet your daily needs.

Stay Hydrated: Drink plenty of water throughout the day to stay hydrated and support optimal body function. Aim for at least 8-10 glasses of water per day, and limit sugary drinks and alcohol, which can contribute to excess calories and dehydration.

In summary, meal planning and prepping are essential for maintaining a healthy and balanced diet while saving time and effort. By following strategies for efficient meal planning and grocery shopping, incorporating batch cooking and freezing meals for convenience, and practicing mindful eating and portion control, you can achieve your health and wellness goals while enjoying delicious and nutritious meals every day.

Nutrisystem:

Definition:

Nutrisystem is a commercial weight loss program that offers pre-packaged meals and snacks delivered directly to customers' homes. The program aims to simplify weight loss by providing portion-controlled, calorie- and nutrient-balanced meals that require minimal preparation. Nutrisystem offers several plans tailored to different dietary preferences and weight loss goals, including basic, core, vegetarian, and diabetic-friendly options. The program also includes support tools such as counseling, online resources, and a mobile app to help participants track progress and stay motivated.

Ingredients:

- Pre-Packaged Meals: Breakfasts, lunches, dinners, and snacks formulated to meet specific calorie and nutritional targets.

- Variety of Foods: Nutrisystem meals and snacks include a range of options such as pasta dishes, pizzas, burgers, soups, salads, and desserts.

- Fruits and Vegetables: Participants are encouraged to supplement Nutrisystem meals with fresh fruits, vegetables, and salads for added fiber, vitamins, and minerals.

- Flex Meals: Nutrisystem offers flexibility with "flex meals," allowing participants to prepare their meals using guidelines provided by the program.

- Snacks: Nutrisystem provides snacks such as bars, shakes, and cookies to help curb hunger between meals.

Instructions/How to Prepare:

1. Choose a Nutrisystem plan based on individual weight loss goals, dietary preferences, and budget.

2. Receive pre-packaged meals and snacks delivered to your doorstep, following the Nutrisystem meal plan and eating schedule.

3. Enjoy Nutrisystem meals and snacks as directed, incorporating fresh fruits, vegetables, and salads as recommended for added nutrition and variety.

4. Supplement Nutrisystem meals with water or other non-caloric beverages to stay hydrated throughout the day.

5. Utilize support tools such as counseling, online resources, and the Nutrisystem app to track progress, access meal plans, and receive personalized guidance and support.

6. Incorporate physical activity into daily routines to complement Nutrisystem's weight loss program and promote overall health and well-being.

7. Practice portion control and mindful eating by savoring each bite and paying attention to hunger and fullness cues.

8. Monitor weight loss progress and adjust Nutrisystem meal plans as needed to achieve and maintain desired results.

9. Continue following Nutrisystem's maintenance plan and lifestyle recommendations to sustain weight loss and promote long-term success.

10. Seek support from the Nutrisystem community, including counselors, fellow participants, and online forums, for motivation, encouragement, and accountability throughout the weight loss journey.

Jenny Craig:

Definition:

Jenny Craig is a commercial weight loss program that combines pre-packaged meals and personalized coaching to help individuals achieve their weight loss goals. The program offers a variety of meal plans tailored to different dietary preferences, including standard, vegetarian, and gluten-free options. Participants receive pre-portioned meals and snacks delivered to their homes or can pick them up at Jenny Craig centers. In addition to meal delivery, Jenny Craig provides one-on-one coaching, support tools, and online resources to help clients develop healthy habits, overcome obstacles, and achieve long-term success.

Ingredients:

- Pre-Packaged Meals: Breakfasts, lunches, dinners, and snacks formulated to meet specific calorie and nutritional targets.

- Variety of Foods: Jenny Craig meals include a range of options such as pasta dishes, pizzas, burgers, soups, salads, and desserts.

- Fresh Additions: Participants are encouraged to supplement Jenny Craig meals with fresh fruits, vegetables, and dairy for added nutrition and variety.

- Snacks: Jenny Craig provides snacks such as bars, shakes, and cookies to help curb hunger between meals.

- Flexibility: Jenny Craig offers flexibility with "Your List," allowing participants to incorporate their favorite foods into their meal plans in moderation.

Instructions/How to Prepare:

1. Enroll in the Jenny Craig program and choose a meal plan based on individual weight loss goals, dietary preferences, and lifestyle.

2. Receive pre-packaged meals and snacks delivered to your home or pick them up at a Jenny Craig center, following the meal plan and eating schedule provided.

3. Enjoy Jenny Craig meals and snacks as directed, incorporating fresh fruits, vegetables, and dairy as recommended for added nutrition and variety.

4. Supplement Jenny Craig meals with water or other non-caloric beverages to stay hydrated throughout the day.

5. Schedule one-on-one coaching sessions with a Jenny Craig consultant to receive personalized support, guidance, and encouragement throughout the weight loss journey.

6. Utilize support tools such as online resources, meal planners, and the Jenny Craig app to track progress, access meal plans, and stay motivated.

7. Incorporate physical activity into daily routines to complement Jenny Craig's weight loss program and promote overall health and well-being.

8. Practice portion control and mindful eating by savoring each bite and paying attention to hunger and fullness cues.

9. Monitor weight loss progress and adjust meal plans as needed to achieve and maintain desired results.

10. Continue following Jenny Craig's maintenance plan and lifestyle recommendations to sustain weight loss and promote long-term success.

SlimFast Diet:

Definition:

The SlimFast Diet is a popular commercial weight loss program that revolves around meal replacement shakes, bars, and snacks.

It offers a structured plan designed to help individuals lose weight by replacing two meals a day with SlimFast products and enjoying one sensible meal and three low-calorie snacks. The program provides portion-controlled, calorie-controlled meals and encourages participants to follow a balanced diet, incorporating fruits, vegetables, lean proteins, and whole grains alongside SlimFast products. Additionally, SlimFast offers support tools, online resources, and a community for motivation and accountability.

Ingredients:

- SlimFast Shakes: Meal replacement shakes available in various flavors, formulated to provide essential nutrients and promote satiety.

- SlimFast Bars: Meal replacement bars available in different flavors, offering a convenient and portable option for on-the-go nutrition.

- SlimFast Snacks: Low-calorie snacks such as snack bars, chips, and crisps designed to satisfy hunger between meals.

Instructions/How to Prepare:

1. Choose a SlimFast plan based on individual weight loss goals, dietary preferences, and lifestyle.

2. Replace two meals a day with SlimFast shakes or bars, enjoying one sensible meal and three low-calorie snacks.

3. Follow the SlimFast meal plan and eating schedule, incorporating fruits, vegetables, lean proteins, and whole grains into sensible meals and snacks.

4. Drink plenty of water throughout the day to stay hydrated and promote overall health and well-being.

5. Utilize support tools such as online resources, meal planners, and the SlimFast app to track progress, access meal plans, and stay motivated.

6. Incorporate physical activity into daily routines to complement the SlimFast weight loss program and promote overall fitness and well-being.

7. Practice portion control and mindful eating by paying attention to hunger and fullness cues and savoring each bite.

8. Monitor weight loss progress and adjust meal plans as needed to achieve and maintain desired results.

9. Continue following the SlimFast maintenance plan and lifestyle recommendations to sustain weight loss and promote long-term success.

10. Seek support from the SlimFast community, including counselors, fellow participants, and online forums, for motivation, encouragement, and accountability throughout the weight loss journey.

Volumetrics Diet:

Definition:

The Volumetrics Diet, developed by Barbara Rolls, PhD, emphasizes eating high-volume, low-calorie foods to promote satiety and weight loss. It focuses on consuming foods that are low in energy density (calories per gram) but high in volume, such as fruits, vegetables, whole grains, and lean proteins. By emphasizing foods with high water content, fiber, and nutrients, the Volumetrics Diet aims to help individuals feel full and satisfied while consuming fewer calories. The diet offers flexibility and variety, allowing participants to enjoy a wide range of foods while still achieving weight loss goals.

Ingredients:

- Fruits: Berries, apples, oranges, bananas, mangoes, melons, etc.

- Vegetables: Leafy greens, broccoli, cauliflower, bell peppers, carrots, onions, etc.

- Whole Grains: Brown rice, quinoa, oats, barley, whole wheat bread, whole grain pasta.

- Lean Proteins: Chicken, turkey, fish, seafood, tofu, tempeh, lean cuts of beef or pork.

- Healthy Fats: Avocado, nuts, seeds, olive oil.

- Low-Calorie Foods: Soups, salads, broth-based dishes, fruits, vegetables, and foods with high water content and low energy density.

Instructions/How to Prepare:

1. Familiarize yourself with the concept of energy density and how it influences food choices and portion sizes.

2. Focus on consuming foods that are low in energy density, such as fruits, vegetables, whole grains, and lean proteins, as the foundation of meals and snacks.

3. Prioritize water-rich foods like soups, salads, and broth-based dishes to increase meal volume without adding extra calories.

4. Incorporate fiber-rich foods such as fruits, vegetables, whole grains, and legumes to promote satiety and support digestive health.

5. Use portion control techniques such as measuring food portions, using smaller plates, and being mindful of serving sizes to manage calorie intake.

6. Be strategic with meal planning and food choices, opting for nutrient-dense foods that provide essential vitamins, minerals, and antioxidants.

7. Include a variety of flavors, textures, and colors in meals to enhance satisfaction and enjoyment.

8. Practice mindful eating by paying attention to hunger and fullness cues, eating slowly, and savoring each bite.

9. Stay hydrated by drinking plenty of water throughout the day, as thirst can sometimes be mistaken for hunger.

10. Monitor weight loss progress and adjust meal plans as needed to achieve and maintain desired results while incorporating lifelong habits for long-term health and well-being.

SparkPeople Diet:

Definition:

The SparkPeople Diet is an online weight loss and wellness program that offers tools, resources, and support for individuals looking to achieve their health and fitness goals. The program provides personalized meal plans, workout routines, tracking tools, and a supportive community to help participants make sustainable lifestyle changes. The SparkPeople Diet focuses on a balanced approach to nutrition, exercise, and behavior change, emphasizing portion control, mindful eating, and regular physical activity. It encourages participants to set realistic goals, track progress, and celebrate successes along the way.

Ingredients:

- Balanced Meals: SparkPeople provides personalized meal plans tailored to individual dietary preferences, calorie needs, and weight loss goals.

- Nutrient-Dense Foods: Participants are encouraged to incorporate a variety of fruits, vegetables, whole grains, lean proteins, and healthy fats into their meals and snacks.

- Portion Control: SparkPeople emphasizes portion control techniques such as measuring food portions, using smaller plates, and being mindful of serving sizes to manage calorie intake.

- Exercise Routines: SparkPeople offers workout routines and fitness videos for participants to incorporate regular physical activity into their daily routines.

- Tracking Tools: SparkPeople provides tracking tools for food intake, exercise, weight loss progress, and other health metrics to help participants stay accountable and monitor their success.

- Supportive Community: SparkPeople offers a supportive online community where participants can connect with others, share experiences, and receive encouragement and motivation.

Instructions/How to Prepare:

1. Sign up for the SparkPeople program and create a personalized profile, including information about dietary preferences, weight loss goals, and activity level.

2. Receive personalized meal plans, workout routines, and tracking tools based on individual needs and goals.

3. Follow the SparkPeople meal plan, incorporating a variety of nutrient-dense foods such as fruits, vegetables, whole grains, lean proteins, and healthy fats into meals and snacks.

4. Practice portion control by measuring food portions, using smaller plates, and being mindful of serving sizes to manage calorie intake.

5. Incorporate regular physical activity into daily routines, following SparkPeople workout routines and fitness videos or engaging in other forms of exercise that are enjoyable and sustainable.

6. Use SparkPeople tracking tools to monitor food intake, exercise, weight loss progress, and other health metrics, staying accountable and motivated along the way.

7. Engage with the SparkPeople community, connecting with others, sharing experiences, and receiving encouragement and support throughout the weight loss journey.

8. Be patient and consistent, recognizing that weight loss and lifestyle changes take time and effort, and celebrating successes along the way.

9. Adjust meal plans, workout routines, and goals as needed based on progress and feedback, staying flexible and adaptable to individual needs and preferences.

10. Embrace a lifelong commitment to health and wellness, incorporating healthy habits into daily life and continuing to strive for improvement and success.

CHAPTER 11

DIET FOR DIABETES

Glycemic Load Diet:

Definition:

The Glycemic Load Diet focuses on managing blood sugar levels by selecting foods based on their glycemic load, which takes into account both the quality and quantity of carbohydrates in a serving of food. The diet aims to minimize blood sugar spikes and promote stable energy levels by emphasizing foods with a low glycemic load, such as fruits, vegetables, whole grains, lean proteins, and healthy fats. It encourages portion control, balanced meals, and mindful eating to support overall health and well-being.

Ingredients:

- Low-Glycemic Foods: Fruits, vegetables, whole grains, legumes, nuts, seeds, lean proteins, and healthy fats.

- High-Fiber Foods: Foods high in fiber such as fruits, vegetables, whole grains, legumes, nuts, and seeds can help slow the absorption of carbohydrates and promote satiety.

- Healthy Fats: Avocado, nuts, seeds, olive oil, fatty fish (salmon, mackerel, sardines) provide essential nutrients and help balance blood sugar levels.

- Lean Proteins: Chicken, turkey, fish, seafood, tofu, tempeh, lean cuts of beef or pork provide satiety and support muscle health.

- Portion-Controlled Carbohydrates: Portion control is emphasized to manage carbohydrate intake and prevent blood sugar spikes.

Instructions/How to Prepare:

1. Understand the concept of glycemic load and how it influences blood sugar levels and overall health.

2. Choose foods with a low glycemic load, such as fruits, vegetables, whole grains, legumes, nuts, seeds, lean proteins, and healthy fats, as the foundation of meals and snacks.

3. Emphasize high-fiber foods to promote satiety, stabilize blood sugar levels, and support digestive health.

4. Incorporate healthy fats into meals and snacks to balance blood sugar levels and promote feelings of fullness and satisfaction.

5. Include lean proteins in meals to provide essential nutrients, promote muscle health, and support satiety.

6. Practice portion control by measuring food portions, using smaller plates, and being mindful of serving sizes to manage carbohydrate intake.

7. Be mindful of meal timing and spacing to prevent blood sugar spikes and maintain stable energy levels throughout the day.

8. Monitor blood sugar levels regularly, especially for individuals with diabetes or insulin resistance, and adjust dietary choices as needed to achieve and maintain optimal blood sugar control.

9. Stay hydrated by drinking plenty of water throughout the day to support overall health and well-being.

10. Seek guidance from a healthcare professional or registered dietitian experienced in glycemic load and blood sugar management for personalized recommendations and support.

Low-Protein Diet:

Definition:

A low-protein diet is a dietary approach that restricts the intake of protein-rich foods, often for medical reasons. It may be prescribed for individuals with certain kidney conditions, liver disease, or metabolic disorders that impair protein metabolism. The diet typically limits high-protein foods such as meat, poultry, fish, eggs, dairy products, and legumes while allowing moderate consumption of low-protein foods such as fruits, vegetables, grains, and fats. The goal of a low-protein diet is to reduce the workload on the kidneys and liver, manage symptoms, and slow the progression of underlying medical conditions.

Ingredients:

- Low-Protein Foods: Fruits, vegetables, grains, fats, and oils are typically allowed in moderate amounts on a low-protein diet.

- Limited Protein Sources: Protein-rich foods such as meat, poultry, fish, eggs, dairy products, and legumes are restricted or limited in portion size.

- Protein-Free Foods: Certain foods may be completely avoided on a low-protein diet, especially those with high protein content.

- Fluids: Adequate hydration is important on a low-protein diet, so drinking water and other low-protein beverages is encouraged.

Instructions/How to Prepare:

1. Consult with a healthcare professional or registered dietitian to determine if a low-protein diet is appropriate for your medical condition and health needs.

2. Receive personalized guidance on the recommended daily intake of protein, as well as specific dietary restrictions and allowances.

3. Identify high-protein foods to limit or avoid, including meat, poultry, fish, eggs, dairy products, and legumes.

4. Plan meals and snacks that emphasize low-protein foods such as fruits, vegetables, grains, and fats while limiting protein-rich ingredients.

5. Use portion control techniques to manage protein intake and ensure compliance with dietary recommendations.

6. Explore alternative protein sources that are lower in protein content, such as tofu, tempeh, seitan, and certain grains and vegetables.

7. Monitor symptoms and adjust dietary choices as needed based on individual tolerance and response to the low-protein diet.

8. Stay hydrated by drinking plenty of water throughout the day, as adequate fluid intake is important for kidney function and overall health.

9. Consider working with a registered dietitian experienced in medical nutrition therapy to develop a customized meal plan and receive ongoing support and guidance.

10. Regularly follow up with healthcare providers to assess progress, monitor kidney function, and adjust dietary recommendations as needed.

The Fast Diet (5:2 Diet):

Definition:

The Fast Diet, also known as the 5:2 Diet, is a popular intermittent fasting approach that involves alternating between regular eating days and fasting days. On fasting days, individuals restrict calorie intake to a quarter of their usual daily intake, typically around 500-600 calories for women and 600-800 calories for men. On non-fasting days, individuals eat normally without calorie restriction. The Fast Diet is believed to promote weight loss, improve metabolic health, and provide other potential health benefits by inducing a state of mild calorie restriction and metabolic adaptation.

Ingredients:

- Regular Eating Days: On non-fasting days, individuals can eat a balanced diet that includes a variety of foods such as fruits, vegetables, whole grains, lean proteins, and healthy fats.

- Fasting Days: On fasting days, individuals consume a limited number of calories, typically from low-calorie foods such as vegetables, fruits, lean proteins, and small amounts of grains and fats.

- Fluids: Adequate hydration is important on fasting days, so drinking water, herbal tea, and other non-caloric beverages is encouraged.

Instructions/How to Prepare:

1. Determine fasting days and non-fasting days based on personal preferences, lifestyle, and schedule.

2. Plan meals and snacks for non-fasting days that provide balanced nutrition and meet individual dietary preferences and calorie needs.

3. On fasting days, consume a limited number of calories, typically around 500-600 calories for women and 600-800 calories for men, spread throughout the day.

4. Choose low-calorie foods that provide satiety and essential nutrients, such as vegetables, fruits, lean proteins, and small amounts of grains and fats.

5. Practice portion control and mindful eating on both fasting and non-fasting days to manage calorie intake and support overall health and well-being.

6. Stay hydrated by drinking plenty of water throughout the day, especially on fasting days when calorie intake is restricted.

7. Consider experimenting with different fasting schedules, such as alternate-day fasting or modified fasting, to find what works best for individual preferences and goals.

8. Be patient and flexible, recognizing that intermittent fasting may take time to adapt to and may not be suitable for everyone.

9. Monitor hunger, energy levels, and overall well-being throughout the fasting period, adjusting dietary choices and fasting schedules as needed.

10. Consult with a healthcare professional or registered dietitian before starting the Fast Diet, especially if you have underlying health conditions or concerns about fasting.

The Warrior Diet:

Definition:

The Warrior Diet is an intermittent fasting approach that involves extended periods of fasting followed by short eating windows. Inspired by ancient warrior cultures, this diet encourages individuals to fast for approximately 20 hours each day and consume one large meal during a 4-hour "overeating" window in the evening. During the fasting period, individuals are encouraged to consume small amounts of raw fruits, vegetables, and non-caloric beverages to support hydration and provide minimal energy. The Warrior Diet is believed to promote fat loss, improve metabolic health, and increase mental clarity and focus by aligning eating patterns with natural circadian rhythms.

Ingredients:

- Fasting Period: During the fasting period, individuals consume small amounts of raw fruits, vegetables, and non-caloric beverages such as water, herbal tea, or black coffee.
- Overeating Window: During the overeating window, individuals consume one large meal that includes a variety of nutrient-dense foods such as lean proteins, whole grains,

fruits, vegetables, healthy fats, and dairy or dairy alternatives.

Instructions/How to Prepare:

1. Determine fasting and eating windows based on personal preferences, lifestyle, and schedule.

2. Start the day with hydration by drinking water, herbal tea, or black coffee during the fasting period to support overall health and well-being.

3. Consume small amounts of raw fruits and vegetables throughout the fasting period to help manage hunger and provide essential nutrients.

4. Break the fast with a large, nutrient-dense meal during the overeating window, incorporating a variety of foods such as lean proteins, whole grains, fruits, vegetables, healthy fats, and dairy or dairy alternatives.

5. Practice mindful eating during the overeating window, focusing on hunger and fullness cues and savoring each bite of food.

6. Stay hydrated throughout the day by drinking plenty of water and other non-caloric beverages to support hydration and overall health.

7. Experiment with different meal compositions and timing strategies to find what works best for individual preferences and goals.

8. Listen to your body and adjust eating patterns as needed based on hunger, energy levels, and overall well-being.

9. Be patient and flexible, recognizing that intermittent fasting may take time to adapt to and may not be suitable for everyone.

10. Consult with a healthcare professional or registered dietitian before starting the Warrior Diet, especially if you have underlying health conditions or concerns about fasting.

The Blood Sugar Solution Diet:

Definition:

The Blood Sugar Solution Diet, developed by Dr. Mark Hyman, is a comprehensive approach to managing blood sugar levels and promoting overall health and well-being. It focuses on reducing inflammation, balancing blood sugar, and optimizing metabolism through dietary changes, lifestyle modifications, and targeted supplementation. The diet emphasizes whole, nutrient-dense foods that support stable blood sugar levels, such as non-starchy vegetables, lean proteins, healthy fats, and low-glycemic carbohydrates. It also encourages individuals to eliminate processed foods, refined sugars, artificial additives, and other inflammatory substances from their diet to reduce insulin resistance and improve metabolic function.

Ingredients:

- Whole Foods: Non-starchy vegetables, leafy greens, lean proteins, nuts, seeds, legumes, whole grains, healthy fats, and low-glycemic fruits are emphasized on The Blood Sugar Solution Diet.

- Nutrient-Dense Foods: Foods rich in essential nutrients, vitamins, minerals, and antioxidants are prioritized to support overall health and well-being.

- Elimination of Processed Foods: Processed foods, refined sugars, artificial additives, trans fats, and other inflammatory substances are eliminated or minimized to reduce inflammation and support metabolic health.

- Hydration: Adequate hydration is important on The Blood Sugar Solution Diet, so drinking water, herbal tea, and other non-caloric beverages is encouraged.

Instructions/How to Prepare:

1. Familiarize yourself with the principles of The Blood Sugar Solution Diet, including recommendations for food choices, portion sizes, meal timing, and lifestyle habits.

2. Stock your kitchen with whole, nutrient-dense foods such as non-starchy vegetables, leafy greens, lean proteins, nuts, seeds, legumes, whole grains, healthy fats, and low-glycemic fruits.

3. Plan meals and snacks that prioritize whole foods and balance macronutrients to support stable blood sugar levels and optimize metabolism.

4. Focus on eating a variety of colors, flavors, and textures in meals to ensure a diverse intake of nutrients and promote satiety and enjoyment.

5. Minimize or eliminate processed foods, refined sugars, artificial additives, trans fats, and other inflammatory substances from your diet to reduce inflammation and support metabolic health.

6. Pay attention to portion sizes and practice mindful eating by listening to hunger and fullness cues, eating slowly, and savoring each bite.

7. Stay hydrated by drinking plenty of water throughout the day to support overall health and well-being.

8. Incorporate regular physical activity into your daily routine to enhance metabolic function, support weight management, and promote overall fitness and well-being.

9. Monitor blood sugar levels regularly, especially for individuals with diabetes or insulin resistance, and adjust dietary choices as needed to achieve and maintain optimal blood sugar control.

10. Consult with a healthcare professional or registered dietitian before starting The Blood Sugar Solution Diet, especially if you have underlying health conditions or concerns about dietary changes.

Mediterranean Diet:

Definition:

The Mediterranean diet is inspired by the traditional dietary patterns of countries bordering the Mediterranean Sea. It emphasizes whole, minimally processed foods such as fruits, vegetables, whole grains, nuts, seeds, legumes, fish, and olive oil. It limits red meat and sweets, while encouraging moderate consumption of dairy products, poultry, and eggs.

Ingredients:

- Fruits: Berries, apples, oranges, grapes, etc.
- Vegetables: Spinach, tomatoes, peppers, onions, etc.
- Whole Grains: Whole wheat bread, brown rice, quinoa, oats, etc.
- Nuts and Seeds: Almonds, walnuts, flaxseeds, chia seeds, etc.

- Legumes: Chickpeas, lentils, beans, etc.
- Fish and Seafood: Salmon, tuna, shrimp, etc.
- Olive Oil: Extra virgin olive oil for cooking and dressing.
- Herbs and Spices: Basil, oregano, garlic, cumin, etc.

Instructions/How to Prepare:

9. Base meals around plant-based foods like fruits, vegetables, whole grains, and legumes.
10. Use olive oil as the primary source of fat for cooking and dressing salads.
11. Incorporate fish and seafood into your diet regularly, aiming for at least two servings per week.
12. Enjoy moderate amounts of poultry, eggs, and dairy products, such as yogurt and cheese.
13. Limit red meat consumption to a few times per month.
14. Snack on nuts and seeds for a healthy source of fats and protein.
15. Flavor meals with herbs and spices instead of salt.
16. Drink plenty of water and enjoy a moderate amount of red wine if desired (optional).

DASH Diet (Dietary Approaches to Stop Hypertension):

Definition:

The DASH diet is specifically designed to help lower blood pressure and reduce the risk of hypertension. It emphasizes fruits, vegetables, whole grains, and lean proteins while limiting sodium, saturated fats, and sweets.

Ingredients:

- Fruits: Berries, bananas, apples, oranges, etc.
- Vegetables: Leafy greens, carrots, broccoli, bell peppers, etc.
- Whole Grains: Brown rice, whole wheat bread, quinoa, oats, barley, etc.
- Lean Proteins: Chicken breast, turkey, fish, tofu, beans, lentils, etc.
- Dairy: Low-fat or fat-free milk, yogurt, cheese, etc.
- Nuts and Seeds: Almonds, pistachios, sunflower seeds, etc.
- Healthy Fats: Olive oil, avocado, nuts, seeds, etc.

Instructions/How to Prepare:

11. Focus on incorporating plenty of fruits and vegetables into your meals and snacks.
12. Choose whole grains over refined grains whenever possible.

13. Opt for lean proteins such as poultry, fish, tofu, and legumes.

14. Limit high-fat dairy products and opt for low-fat or fat-free options.

15. Include nuts and seeds as snacks or in salads for added nutrients and healthy fats.

16. Use herbs, spices, and citrus juices to flavor foods instead of salt.

17. Avoid processed and high-sodium foods like canned soups, packaged snacks, and fast food.

18. Cook meals at home whenever possible to have better control over ingredients and portion sizes.

19. Aim to limit sweets and sugary beverages, opting for natural sweeteners like fruit when craving something sweet.

20. Stay hydrated by drinking plenty of water throughout the day.

Low-Carb Diet:

Definition:

A low-carb diet involves reducing carbohydrate intake while increasing the consumption of protein and healthy fats. This diet aims to control insulin levels, promote weight loss, and improve overall health by limiting foods high in carbohydrates such as bread, pasta, rice, and sugary snacks.

Ingredients:

- Protein Sources: Meat, poultry, fish, tofu, tempeh, eggs.
- Non-Starchy Vegetables: Leafy greens, broccoli, cauliflower, zucchini, bell peppers.
- Healthy Fats: Avocado, nuts, seeds, olive oil, coconut oil.
- Dairy: Cheese, Greek yogurt, cottage cheese (in moderation).
- Low-Carb Fruits: Berries, avocados, tomatoes, lemons, limes.
- Herbs and Spices: Basil, oregano, garlic, turmeric, cumin.
- Sweeteners (optional): Stevia, erythritol, monk fruit.

Instructions/How to Prepare:

9. Focus on whole, unprocessed foods.
10. Limit carbohydrate intake to around 20-50 grams per day, depending on individual needs and goals.
11. Include protein-rich foods in each meal to promote satiety and muscle maintenance.
12. Fill up on non-starchy vegetables to increase fiber intake and provide essential vitamins and minerals.

13. Incorporate healthy fats into your diet for energy and to keep you feeling full.

14. Be mindful of hidden carbs in sauces, condiments, and processed foods.

15. Drink plenty of water to stay hydrated and support overall health.

16. Experiment with low-carb recipes and meal prep to make adhering to the diet easier and more enjoyable.

Ketogenic Diet (Keto Diet):

Definition:

The ketogenic diet is a very low-carb, high-fat diet that forces the body to enter a state of ketosis, where it primarily burns fat for fuel instead of carbohydrates. This diet has been used for decades to treat epilepsy and has gained popularity for weight loss and improving metabolic health.

Ingredients:

- Healthy Fats: Avocado, coconut oil, olive oil, butter, ghee, fatty fish.

- Protein Sources: Meat, poultry, fish, eggs, tofu, tempeh.

- Non-Starchy Vegetables: Leafy greens, broccoli, cauliflower, zucchini, asparagus.

- Full-Fat Dairy: Cheese, heavy cream, Greek yogurt (in moderation).
- Nuts and Seeds: Macadamia nuts, almonds, chia seeds, flaxseeds.
- Low-Carb Fruits: Berries (in moderation), avocado.
- Herbs and Spices: Turmeric, ginger, cinnamon, garlic, thyme.
- Sweeteners (in moderation): Stevia, erythritol, monk fruit.

Instructions/How to Prepare:

9. Keep carbohydrate intake extremely low, typically below 20-50 grams per day to induce and maintain ketosis.

10. Consume moderate amounts of protein, as excessive protein intake can potentially hinder ketosis.

11. Base meals around healthy fats, such as avocados, olive oil, and fatty fish.

12. Incorporate non-starchy vegetables to provide essential nutrients and fiber while keeping carbohydrate intake low.

13. Be mindful of hidden carbs in foods and beverages, including sauces, dressings, and flavored beverages.

14. Stay hydrated by drinking plenty of water, as dehydration can occur more easily on a ketogenic diet.

15. Monitor ketone levels using urine strips, blood tests, or breath meters if desired, to ensure you are in ketosis.

16. Experiment with keto-friendly recipes and meal planning to maintain variety and enjoyment while following the diet.

Plant-Based Diet:

Definition:

A plant-based diet primarily consists of foods derived from plants, such as fruits, vegetables, grains, nuts, seeds, and legumes. It emphasizes whole, minimally processed foods while minimizing or eliminating animal products. The focus is on incorporating a variety of plant foods to promote health and well-being.

Ingredients:

- Fruits: Berries, apples, oranges, bananas, etc.
- Vegetables: Leafy greens, broccoli, carrots, bell peppers, etc.
- Whole Grains: Brown rice, quinoa, oats, barley, whole wheat bread, etc.
- Legumes: Chickpeas, lentils, black beans, kidney beans, etc.
- Nuts and Seeds: Almonds, walnuts, chia seeds, flaxseeds, pumpkin seeds, etc.

- Plant-Based Proteins: Tofu, tempeh, seitan, edamame, plant-based protein powders, etc.

- Healthy Fats: Avocado, olive oil, coconut oil, nuts, seeds, etc.

Instructions/How to Prepare:

11. Base meals around a variety of whole plant foods, including fruits, vegetables, whole grains, legumes, nuts, and seeds.

12. Incorporate a rainbow of colorful fruits and vegetables to ensure a diverse array of nutrients.

13. Include plant-based proteins such as tofu, tempeh, and legumes in meals to meet protein needs.

14. Choose whole grains over refined grains for added fiber and nutrients.

15. Experiment with different cooking methods, such as steaming, roasting, sautéing, and grilling, to enhance flavor and texture.

16. Use herbs, spices, and condiments to add flavor to dishes without relying on animal products.

17. Be mindful of nutrient needs, particularly vitamin B12, vitamin D, omega-3 fatty acids, iron, calcium, and zinc, and consider supplementation if necessary.

18. Stay hydrated by drinking plenty of water throughout the day.

19. Plan balanced meals and snacks to ensure adequate intake of essential nutrients.

20. Enjoy plant-based alternatives to dairy and meat products, such as plant-based milk, cheese, yogurt, and meat substitutes, if desired.

Vegan Diet:

Definition:

A vegan diet excludes all animal products, including meat, poultry, fish, dairy, eggs, and honey. It is based entirely on plant foods and emphasizes cruelty-free living and environmental sustainability.

Ingredients:

- Fruits: Berries, apples, oranges, mangoes, etc.
- Vegetables: Spinach, kale, tomatoes, onions, mushrooms, etc.
- Whole Grains: Quinoa, brown rice, barley, whole wheat pasta, etc.
- Legumes: Chickpeas, black beans, lentils, kidney beans, etc.

- Nuts and Seeds: Almonds, cashews, sunflower seeds, chia seeds, etc.
- Plant-Based Proteins: Tofu, tempeh, seitan, soy-based meat substitutes, etc.
- Healthy Fats: Avocado, olive oil, coconut oil, nuts, seeds, etc.
- Plant-Based Dairy Alternatives: Almond milk, coconut milk, soy milk, vegan cheese, vegan yogurt, etc.

Instructions/How to Prepare:

11. Build meals around plant foods, including fruits, vegetables, whole grains, legumes, nuts, and seeds.

12. Ensure adequate protein intake by including sources such as tofu, tempeh, legumes, and plant-based meat substitutes.

13. Use plant-based milk, cheese, and yogurt alternatives in place of dairy products.

14. Experiment with vegan cooking techniques and recipes to discover new flavors and textures.

15. Pay attention to nutrient needs, especially vitamin B12, vitamin D, omega-3 fatty acids, iron, calcium, and zinc, and consider supplementation if necessary.

16. Read labels carefully to avoid hidden animal ingredients in processed foods and beverages.

17. Be mindful of cross-contamination when preparing and consuming food to prevent unintentional consumption of animal products.

18. Explore vegan-friendly restaurants and eateries or plan ahead when dining out to ensure vegan options are available.

19. Connect with vegan communities and resources for support, recipe ideas, and lifestyle tips.

20. Embrace the ethical and environmental principles of veganism beyond diet by choosing cruelty-free and sustainable products in other areas of life, such as clothing, cosmetics, and household items.

Vegetarian Diet:

Definition:

A vegetarian diet excludes meat, poultry, and seafood, but includes plant-based foods such as fruits, vegetables, grains, nuts, seeds, and dairy products. There are different variations of vegetarianism, including lacto-vegetarian (includes dairy but not eggs), ovo-vegetarian (includes eggs but not dairy), and lacto-ovo-vegetarian (includes both dairy and eggs).

Ingredients:

- Fruits: Berries, apples, oranges, bananas, etc.
- Vegetables: Leafy greens, broccoli, carrots, bell peppers, etc.
- Whole Grains: Brown rice, quinoa, oats, barley, whole wheat bread, etc.
- Legumes: Chickpeas, lentils, black beans, kidney beans, etc.
- Nuts and Seeds: Almonds, walnuts, chia seeds, flaxseeds, pumpkin seeds, etc.
- Dairy: Milk, yogurt, cheese, butter, etc. (depending on the type of vegetarianism)
- Plant-Based Proteins: Tofu, tempeh, seitan, edamame, etc.
- Healthy Fats: Avocado, olive oil, coconut oil, nuts, seeds, etc.

Instructions/How to Prepare:

11. Base meals around a variety of plant foods, including fruits, vegetables, whole grains, legumes, nuts, and seeds.
12. Incorporate plant-based proteins such as tofu, tempeh, legumes, nuts, and seeds into meals to meet protein needs.

13. Choose whole grains over refined grains for added fiber and nutrients.

14. Experiment with different cooking methods, such as steaming, roasting, sautéing, and grilling, to enhance flavor and texture.

15. Use herbs, spices, and condiments to add flavor to dishes without relying on meat.

16. Be mindful of nutrient needs, especially vitamin B12, vitamin D, omega-3 fatty acids, iron, calcium, and zinc, and consider supplementation if necessary.

17. Stay hydrated by drinking plenty of water throughout the day.

18. Plan balanced meals and snacks to ensure adequate intake of essential nutrients.

19. Explore vegetarian cooking techniques and recipes to discover new flavors and textures.

20. Connect with vegetarian communities and resources for support, recipe ideas, and lifestyle tips.

Atkins Diet:

Definition:

The Atkins diet is a low-carbohydrate, high-fat diet designed for weight loss and improving overall health. It involves reducing carbohydrate intake while increasing the consumption of protein and healthy fats. The diet is divided into four phases: induction, balancing, fine-tuning, and maintenance.

Ingredients:

- Protein Sources: Meat, poultry, fish, eggs, tofu, tempeh, etc.
- Non-Starchy Vegetables: Leafy greens, broccoli, cauliflower, zucchini, bell peppers, etc.
- Healthy Fats: Avocado, olive oil, coconut oil, butter, ghee, fatty fish, etc.
- Full-Fat Dairy (in moderation): Cheese, Greek yogurt, heavy cream, etc.
- Nuts and Seeds (in moderation): Almonds, walnuts, chia seeds, flaxseeds, etc.
- Low-Carb Fruits (in moderation): Berries, avocados, tomatoes, etc.
- Herbs and Spices: Basil, oregano, garlic, turmeric, cumin, etc.

Instructions/How to Prepare:

11. Start with the induction phase, which restricts carbohydrate intake to 20-25 grams per day for two weeks to induce ketosis.

12. Base meals around protein-rich foods such as meat, poultry, fish, eggs, and tofu.

13. Include non-starchy vegetables to provide essential nutrients and fiber while keeping carbohydrate intake low.

14. Incorporate healthy fats into your diet for energy and to keep you feeling full.

15. Gradually increase carbohydrate intake during the balancing, fine-tuning, and maintenance phases while monitoring weight and overall health.

16. Be mindful of portion sizes and track carbohydrate intake to stay within the recommended limits for each phase.

17. Stay hydrated by drinking plenty of water throughout the day.

18. Experiment with low-carb recipes and meal planning to maintain variety and enjoyment while following the diet.

19. Consider working with a healthcare professional or registered dietitian to personalize the diet plan and ensure nutritional adequacy.

20. Monitor progress and make adjustments as needed to achieve weight loss and health goals.

South Beach Diet:

Definition:

The South Beach Diet is a popular weight-loss program that emphasizes the consumption of lean protein, healthy fats, and low-glycemic carbohydrates. It's divided into three phases: Phase 1, which eliminates most carbs to jump-start weight loss; Phase 2, which reintroduces some carbs while continuing weight loss; and Phase 3, which focuses on maintaining weight loss with a balanced diet.

Ingredients:

- Lean Proteins: Chicken breast, turkey, fish, seafood, lean cuts of beef and pork.

- Healthy Fats: Olive oil, avocado, nuts, seeds, fatty fish like salmon and mackerel.

- Low-Glycemic Carbohydrates: Non-starchy vegetables (e.g., spinach, broccoli, cauliflower), whole grains (e.g., quinoa, barley), legumes (e.g., beans, lentils).

- Low-Fat Dairy: Greek yogurt, skim milk, low-fat cheese.

Instructions/How to Prepare:

4. Phase 1: Eliminate most carbohydrates, including fruits, grains, and starchy vegetables. Focus on lean proteins, non-starchy vegetables, and healthy fats. Drink plenty of water and avoid processed foods and added sugars.

5. Phase 2: Gradually reintroduce some carbohydrates, such as fruits and whole grains, while continuing to prioritize lean proteins and healthy fats. Monitor portion sizes and continue to avoid refined sugars and processed foods.

6. Phase 3: Transition to a balanced diet that includes a variety of foods from all food groups. Focus on portion control, mindful eating, and regular physical activity to maintain weight loss and overall health.

Paleo Diet:

Definition:

The Paleo diet, also known as the Paleolithic or caveman diet, is based on the presumed diet of ancient humans during the Paleolithic era. It emphasizes whole foods that would have been available to our hunter-gatherer ancestors, such as lean meats, fish, fruits, vegetables, nuts, and seeds, while excluding processed foods, grains, legumes, and dairy products.

Ingredients:

- Lean Meats: Beef, chicken, turkey, pork, lamb, etc.
- Fish and Seafood: Salmon, trout, shrimp, shellfish, etc.
- Fruits: Berries, apples, oranges, bananas, etc.
- Vegetables: Leafy greens, broccoli, carrots, peppers, onions, etc.
- Nuts and Seeds: Almonds, walnuts, cashews, sunflower seeds, etc.
- Healthy Fats: Avocado, olive oil, coconut oil, ghee.
- Herbs and Spices: Basil, oregano, garlic, turmeric, cinnamon, etc.

Instructions/How to Prepare:

11. Base meals around lean proteins, including meat, fish, and seafood.

12. Incorporate a variety of colorful fruits and vegetables for essential vitamins, minerals, and fiber.

13. Include nuts and seeds as snacks or to add texture and flavor to meals.

14. Use healthy fats like olive oil, avocado, and coconut oil for cooking and dressing.

15. Avoid processed foods, grains, legumes, dairy products, refined sugars, and artificial additives.

16. Experiment with cooking methods such as grilling, baking, and sautéing to enhance flavor and texture.

17. Stay hydrated by drinking plenty of water throughout the day.

18. Listen to your body's hunger and fullness cues and eat mindfully.

19. Be aware of portion sizes and adjust based on individual energy needs and activity levels.

20. Focus on whole, nutrient-dense foods and prioritize quality over quantity.

Whole30 Diet:

Definition:

The Whole30 diet is a 30-day elimination diet designed to reset your body and identify potential food sensitivities. It involves removing certain food groups known to cause inflammation and digestive issues, such as sugar, grains, dairy, legumes, and processed foods, for 30 days. After the elimination period, foods are gradually reintroduced to identify which ones may be causing adverse reactions.

Ingredients:

- Protein Sources: Meat, poultry, fish, seafood, eggs.
- Vegetables: Leafy greens, cruciferous vegetables, peppers, squash, etc.
- Fruits: Berries, apples, oranges, bananas, etc.
- Healthy Fats: Avocado, olive oil, coconut oil, nuts, seeds.
- Herbs and Spices: Basil, oregano, garlic, turmeric, cinnamon, etc.

Instructions/How to Prepare:

11. Eliminate sugar, grains, dairy, legumes, and processed foods from your diet for 30 days.
12. Base meals around protein sources, including meat, poultry, fish, seafood, and eggs.
13. Include a variety of vegetables for essential vitamins, minerals, and fiber.
14. Incorporate fruits as snacks or to add natural sweetness to meals.
15. Use healthy fats like avocado, olive oil, and coconut oil for cooking and dressing.
16. Experiment with herbs and spices to enhance flavor without added sugars or artificial additives.

17. Be mindful of hidden sources of sugar and processed ingredients in condiments and packaged foods.

18. Read labels carefully and opt for whole, minimally processed foods.

19. Stay hydrated by drinking plenty of water throughout the day.

20. After the 30-day elimination period, reintroduce eliminated foods one at a time and monitor for any adverse reactions or changes in symptoms.

Low-Glycemic Index Diet:

Definition:

The Low-Glycemic Index (GI) diet focuses on consuming foods that have a low glycemic index, which means they cause a slower and more gradual increase in blood sugar levels. This diet can help stabilize blood sugar, improve insulin sensitivity, and promote weight loss. Foods with a low GI typically include non-starchy vegetables, whole grains, lean proteins, and healthy fats.

Ingredients:

- Non-Starchy Vegetables: Leafy greens, broccoli, cauliflower, peppers, carrots, etc.
- Whole Grains: Quinoa, barley, bulgur, oats, brown rice, etc.

- Lean Proteins: Chicken breast, turkey, fish, tofu, tempeh, beans, lentils.

- Healthy Fats: Avocado, olive oil, nuts, seeds, fatty fish like salmon.

- Low-Glycemic Fruits (in moderation): Berries, apples, oranges, pears, etc.

- Herbs and Spices: Basil, oregano, garlic, turmeric, cinnamon, etc.

Instructions/How to Prepare:

11. Choose whole, minimally processed foods with a low glycemic index.

12. Base meals around non-starchy vegetables, whole grains, and lean proteins.

13. Incorporate healthy fats like avocado, olive oil, nuts, and seeds for satiety and flavor.

14. Limit high-glycemic foods such as refined grains, sugary snacks, and sweetened beverages.

15. Include low-glycemic fruits in moderation, focusing on berries, apples, and citrus fruits.

16. Be mindful of portion sizes and avoid overeating, even with low-GI foods.

17. Experiment with cooking methods such as steaming, roasting, and sautéing to enhance flavor and texture.

18. Eat balanced meals that combine protein, carbohydrates, and healthy fats to promote satiety and stabilize blood sugar levels.

19. Monitor blood sugar levels if necessary and adjust your diet accordingly.

20. Stay hydrated by drinking plenty of water throughout the day.

Low-Fat Diet:

Definition:

A low-fat diet is characterized by reducing the intake of dietary fats, particularly saturated fats and trans fats, to promote heart health, manage weight, and reduce the risk of certain chronic diseases such as cardiovascular disease. This diet typically involves limiting foods high in fat and choosing lean protein sources, whole grains, fruits, vegetables, and low-fat dairy products.

Ingredients:

- Lean Proteins: Skinless poultry, lean cuts of beef and pork, fish, tofu, tempeh, legumes.

- Whole Grains: Brown rice, quinoa, barley, whole wheat bread, oats, whole grain pasta.

- Fruits: Berries, apples, oranges, bananas, grapes, etc.

- Vegetables: Leafy greens, broccoli, carrots, bell peppers, tomatoes, etc.

- Low-Fat or Fat-Free Dairy: Skim milk, low-fat yogurt, reduced-fat cheese.

- Healthy Fats (in moderation): Avocado, nuts, seeds, olive oil.

Instructions/How to Prepare:

11. Choose lean protein sources such as poultry, fish, tofu, and legumes instead of high-fat meats.

12. Opt for whole grains like brown rice, quinoa, and whole wheat bread over refined grains.

13. Include a variety of fruits and vegetables in your meals and snacks for added vitamins, minerals, and fiber.

14. Select low-fat or fat-free dairy products to reduce saturated fat intake.

15. Limit added fats and oils, and use healthier cooking methods such as baking, grilling, steaming, or boiling.

16. Be mindful of portion sizes to avoid overconsumption of calories, even with low-fat foods.

17. Read food labels to identify hidden sources of fat and choose lower-fat options when available.

18. Incorporate healthy fats like avocado, nuts, and olive oil in moderation for flavor and satiety.

19. Stay hydrated by drinking plenty of water throughout the day.

20. Focus on overall dietary patterns rather than just reducing fat intake, and aim for a balanced diet that includes a variety of nutrient-dense foods.

The Insulin-Resistance Diet:

Definition:

The Insulin-Resistance Diet is a dietary approach aimed at managing insulin resistance, a condition in which cells become less responsive to the effects of insulin, leading to elevated blood sugar levels. This diet focuses on regulating blood sugar levels, improving insulin sensitivity, and promoting overall health and well-being. It emphasizes whole, nutrient-dense foods that have a minimal impact on blood sugar levels, such as non-starchy vegetables, lean proteins, healthy fats, and high-fiber carbohydrates. The Insulin-Resistance Diet also encourages regular physical activity, stress management, and lifestyle modifications to support metabolic health.

Ingredients:

- Whole Foods: Non-starchy vegetables, leafy greens, lean proteins, nuts, seeds, legumes, whole grains, healthy fats, and low-glycemic fruits are emphasized on The Insulin-Resistance Diet.

- High-Fiber Carbohydrates: Carbohydrates with a high fiber content, such as whole grains, legumes, fruits, and vegetables, are preferred to support stable blood sugar levels and promote satiety.

- Lean Proteins: Lean sources of protein, including poultry, fish, tofu, tempeh, legumes, and low-fat dairy products, are prioritized to support muscle health and metabolic function.

- Healthy Fats: Monounsaturated and polyunsaturated fats from sources such as avocados, nuts, seeds, olive oil, and fatty fish are encouraged to provide essential nutrients and support cardiovascular health.

- Low-Glycemic Foods: Foods with a low glycemic index, which have a minimal impact on blood sugar levels, are favored on The Insulin-Resistance Diet to help regulate insulin levels and prevent spikes and crashes in blood sugar.

Instructions/How to Prepare:

1. Educate yourself about insulin resistance and how dietary and lifestyle factors can influence blood sugar levels and insulin sensitivity.

2. Stock your kitchen with whole, nutrient-dense foods such as non-starchy vegetables, leafy greens, lean proteins, nuts, seeds, legumes, whole grains, healthy fats, and low-glycemic fruits.

3. Plan meals and snacks that prioritize whole foods and balance macronutrients to support stable blood sugar levels and improve insulin sensitivity.

4. Focus on eating a variety of colors, flavors, and textures in meals to ensure a diverse intake of nutrients and promote satiety and enjoyment.

5. Choose high-fiber carbohydrates such as whole grains, legumes, fruits, and vegetables to slow the absorption of sugar into the bloodstream and prevent spikes in blood sugar levels.

6. Incorporate lean sources of protein into meals and snacks to support muscle health, promote satiety, and stabilize blood sugar levels.

7. Include healthy fats from sources such as avocados, nuts, seeds, olive oil, and fatty fish to provide essential nutrients and support cardiovascular health.

8. Minimize or eliminate processed foods, refined sugars, artificial additives, trans fats, and other inflammatory substances from your diet to reduce inflammation and improve metabolic health.

9. Pay attention to portion sizes and practice mindful eating by listening to hunger and fullness cues, eating slowly, and savoring each bite.

10. Stay hydrated by drinking plenty of water throughout the day to support overall health and well-being.

The Sugar Busters Diet:

Definition:

The Sugar Busters Diet is a low-glycemic approach to eating that aims to control blood sugar levels and promote weight loss by minimizing the consumption of high-glycemic carbohydrates and sugars. It emphasizes whole, nutrient-dense foods that have a minimal impact on blood sugar levels, such as non-starchy vegetables, lean proteins, healthy fats, and low-glycemic carbohydrates. The Sugar Busters Diet also encourages portion control, regular physical activity, and lifestyle modifications to support metabolic health and overall well-being.

Ingredients:

- Whole Foods: Non-starchy vegetables, leafy greens, lean proteins, nuts, seeds, legumes, whole grains, healthy fats, and low-glycemic fruits are emphasized on The Sugar Busters Diet.

- Low-Glycemic Carbohydrates: Carbohydrates with a low glycemic index, such as whole grains, legumes, fruits, and vegetables, are preferred to help regulate blood sugar levels and prevent spikes and crashes in blood sugar.

- Lean Proteins: Lean sources of protein, including poultry, fish, tofu, tempeh, legumes, and low-fat dairy products, are prioritized to support muscle health and metabolic function.

- Healthy Fats: Monounsaturated and polyunsaturated fats from sources such as avocados, nuts, seeds, olive oil, and fatty fish are encouraged to provide essential nutrients and support cardiovascular health.

Instructions/How to Prepare:

1. Familiarize yourself with the principles of The Sugar Busters Diet, including recommendations for food choices, portion sizes, meal timing, and lifestyle habits.

2. Stock your kitchen with whole, nutrient-dense foods such as non-starchy vegetables, leafy greens, lean proteins, nuts, seeds, legumes, whole grains, healthy fats, and low-glycemic fruits.

3. Plan meals and snacks that prioritize whole foods and balance macronutrients to support stable blood sugar levels and improve insulin sensitivity.

4. Focus on eating a variety of colors, flavors, and textures in meals to ensure a diverse intake of nutrients and promote satiety and enjoyment.

5. Choose low-glycemic carbohydrates such as whole grains, legumes, fruits, and vegetables to help regulate blood sugar levels and prevent spikes and crashes in blood sugar.

6. Incorporate lean sources of protein into meals and snacks to support muscle health, promote satiety, and stabilize blood sugar levels.

7. Include healthy fats from sources such as avocados, nuts, seeds, olive oil, and fatty fish to provide essential nutrients and support cardiovascular health.

8. Practice portion control by measuring food portions, using smaller plates, and being mindful of serving sizes to manage calorie intake and support weight loss.

9. Stay hydrated by drinking plenty of water throughout the day to support overall health and well-being.

10. Incorporate regular physical activity into your daily routine to enhance metabolic function, support weight management, and promote overall fitness and well-being.

Here's a 31-day meal plan from "The Diabetic Cookbook for Newly Diagnosed" to help navigate a diabetic-friendly diet:

CHAPTER 12

31 DAYS MEAL PLAN

Week 1:

Day 1:

- Breakfast: Scrambled eggs with sautéed spinach and whole grain toast.
- Lunch: Grilled chicken salad with mixed greens, cherry tomatoes, and a light vinaigrette dressing.
- Dinner: Baked salmon with roasted asparagus and quinoa.

Day 2:

- Breakfast: Greek yogurt parfait with berries and a sprinkle of almonds.
- Lunch: Turkey and avocado wrap with lettuce and tomato on a whole wheat tortilla.
- Dinner: Beef stir-fry with broccoli, bell peppers, and brown rice.

Day 3:

- Breakfast: Oatmeal topped with sliced strawberries and a drizzle of honey.

- Lunch: Tuna salad lettuce wraps with cucumber and carrot sticks.
- Dinner: Baked chicken breast with steamed green beans and mashed sweet potatoes.

Day 4:

- Breakfast: Whole grain toast with mashed avocado and a poached egg.
- Lunch: Mediterranean chickpea salad with cucumber, tomatoes, and feta cheese.
- Dinner: Lentil soup with a side of whole grain bread.

Day 5:

- Breakfast: Smoothie made with spinach, banana, Greek yogurt, and almond milk.
- Lunch: Turkey and cheese roll-ups with whole grain crackers and celery sticks.
- Dinner: Baked cod with lemon and herbs, served with roasted Brussels sprouts.

Day 6:

- Breakfast: Cottage cheese with pineapple chunks and a sprinkle of cinnamon.

- Lunch: Quinoa salad with black beans, corn, cherry tomatoes, and lime dressing.
- Dinner: Grilled shrimp skewers with zucchini noodles and marinara sauce.

Day 7:

- Breakfast: Whole grain waffle with peanut butter and sliced bananas.
- Lunch: Greek salad with feta cheese, olives, cucumber, and bell peppers.
- Dinner: Turkey chili with mixed beans and a side of steamed broccoli.

Week 2:

Day 8:

- Breakfast: Scrambled eggs with diced bell peppers and onions.
- Lunch: Chicken Caesar salad with whole grain croutons.
- Dinner: Baked tofu with stir-fried vegetables and brown rice.

Day 9:

- Breakfast: Yogurt with mixed berries and a sprinkle of granola.

- Lunch: Turkey and avocado whole wheat wrap with lettuce and tomato.
- Dinner: Beef and broccoli stir-fry over cauliflower rice.

Day 10:

- Breakfast: Whole grain toast with mashed avocado and a poached egg.
- Lunch: Mediterranean chickpea salad with cucumber, tomatoes, and olives.
- Dinner: Baked salmon with roasted Brussels sprouts and quinoa.

Day 11:

- Breakfast: Smoothie made with spinach, mango, Greek yogurt, and almond milk.
- Lunch: Turkey and cheese sandwich on whole grain bread with carrot sticks.
- Dinner: Lentil curry with brown rice and steamed spinach.

Day 12:

- Breakfast: Cottage cheese with sliced peaches and a sprinkle of chopped walnuts.
- Lunch: Quinoa tabbouleh with cherry tomatoes and cucumber.

- Dinner: Grilled chicken breast with roasted sweet potatoes and green beans.

Day 13:

- Breakfast: Whole grain waffle with peanut butter and sliced bananas.
- Lunch: Caprese salad with mozzarella, tomatoes, and basil.
- Dinner: Baked cod with lemon and herbs, served with quinoa and steamed broccoli.

Day 14:

- Breakfast: Oatmeal with sliced apples and a sprinkle of cinnamon.
- Lunch: Turkey and cheese roll-ups with whole grain crackers and cucumber slices.
- Dinner: Lentil soup with a side of whole grain bread.

Week 3:

Day 15:

- Breakfast: Scrambled eggs with diced bell peppers and onions.
- Lunch: Chicken Caesar salad with whole grain croutons.
- Dinner: Baked tofu with stir-fried vegetables and brown rice.

Day 16:

- Breakfast: Greek yogurt with sliced peaches and a sprinkle of granola.
- Lunch: Turkey and avocado whole wheat wrap with lettuce and tomato.
- Dinner: Beef and broccoli stir-fry over cauliflower rice.

Day 17:

- Breakfast: Whole grain toast with mashed avocado and a poached egg.
- Lunch: Mediterranean chickpea salad with cucumber, tomatoes, and olives.
- Dinner: Baked salmon with roasted Brussels sprouts and quinoa.

Day 18:

- Breakfast: Smoothie made with spinach, mango, Greek yogurt, and almond milk.
- Lunch: Turkey and cheese sandwich on whole grain bread with carrot sticks.
- Dinner: Lentil curry with brown rice and steamed spinach.

Day 19:

- Breakfast: Cottage cheese with sliced peaches and a sprinkle of chopped walnuts.
- Lunch: Quinoa tabbouleh with cherry tomatoes and cucumber.
- Dinner: Grilled chicken breast with roasted sweet potatoes and green beans.

Day 20:

- Breakfast: Whole grain waffle with peanut butter and sliced bananas.
- Lunch: Caprese salad with mozzarella, tomatoes, and basil.
- Dinner: Baked cod with lemon and herbs, served with quinoa and steamed broccoli.

Day 21:

- Breakfast: Oatmeal with sliced apples and a sprinkle of cinnamon.
- Lunch: Turkey and cheese roll-ups with whole grain crackers and cucumber slices.
- Dinner: Lentil soup with a side of whole grain bread.

Week 4:

Day 22:

- Breakfast: Scrambled eggs with diced bell peppers and onions.
- Lunch: Chicken Caesar salad with whole grain croutons.
- Dinner: Baked tofu with stir-fried vegetables and brown rice.

Day 23:

- Breakfast: Greek yogurt with sliced peaches and a sprinkle of granola.
- Lunch: Turkey and avocado whole wheat wrap with lettuce and tomato.
- Dinner: Beef and broccoli stir-fry over cauliflower rice.

Day 24:

- Breakfast: Whole grain toast with mashed avocado and a poached egg.
- Lunch: Mediterranean chickpea salad with cucumber, tomatoes, and olives.
- Dinner: Baked salmon with roasted Brussels sprouts and quinoa.

Day 25:

- Breakfast: Smoothie made with spinach, mango, Greek yogurt, and almond milk.

- Lunch: Turkey and cheese sandwich on whole grain bread with carrot sticks.

- Dinner: Lentil curry with brown rice and steamed spinach.

Day 26:

- Breakfast: Cottage cheese with sliced peaches and a sprinkle of chopped walnuts.

- Lunch: Quinoa tabbouleh with cherry tomatoes and cucumber.

- Dinner: Grilled chicken breast with roasted sweet potatoes and green beans.

Day 27:

- Breakfast: Whole grain waffle with peanut butter and sliced bananas.

- Lunch: Caprese salad with mozzarella, tomatoes, and basil.

- Dinner: Baked cod with lemon and herbs, served with quinoa and steamed broccoli.

Day 28:

- Breakfast: Oatmeal with sliced apples and a sprinkle of cinnamon.

- Lunch: Turkey and cheese roll-ups with whole grain crackers and cucumber slices.

- Dinner: Lentil soup with a side of whole grain bread.

Day 29:

- Breakfast: Scrambled eggs with diced bell peppers and onions.
- Lunch: Chicken Caesar salad with whole grain croutons.
- Dinner: Baked tofu with stir-fried vegetables and brown rice.

Day 30:

- Breakfast: Greek yogurt with sliced peaches and a sprinkle of granola.
- Lunch: Turkey and avocado whole wheat wrap with lettuce and tomato.
- Dinner: Beef and broccoli stir-fry over cauliflower rice.

Day 31:

- Breakfast: Whole grain toast with mashed avocado and a poached egg.
- Lunch: Mediterranean chickpea salad with cucumber, tomatoes, and olives.
- Dinner: Baked salmon with roasted Brussels sprouts and quinoa.

THE END

www.ingramcontent.com/pod-product-compliance
Lightning Source LLC
Chambersburg PA
CBHW082330220526
45470CB00008B/2461